FOOD ENZYMES
for
Health and Longevity
3rd Edition – Revised and Enlarged

DR. EDWARD HOWELL

introduction by
Victoras Kulvinskas, M.S.

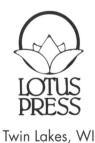

LOTUS
PRESS

Twin Lakes, WI

DISCLAIMER

For information write
Lotus Press, division of Lotus Brands, Inc.,
Box 325, Twin Lakes, WI 53181, USA.
800-824-6396 Website: www.lotuspress.com
Email: lotuspress@lotuspress.com

Revised and Enlarged
3rd Edition 2014.

Published by Lotus Press March 1994
2 3 4 5   99 98 97 96

ISBN: 978-0-9406-7627-5
Library of Congress Catalog Card Number 94-75625

PRINTED IN THE USA

EDITOR'S NOTE

This classic book on the 'Food Enzyme Concept', formulated and developed by Dr. Edward Howell, appeared first in 1946 under the title,' The Status of Food Enzymes in Digestion and Metabolism'. In 1980, it was reissued with the addition of an Interview with the author conducted by noted nutritionist, author and lecturer, Victoras Kulvinskas, M.S.

The present Edition incorporates all the material presented in the 1980 edition of the book, with minor correction and modifications for the sake of clarity. In addition, however, a more recent interview with Dr. Howell has been included, and the previous interview has been retained as an Appendix. For doctors, scientists, and researchers who would like to go to the original sources of the scientific literature which partly helped Dr. Howell develop his, for that time revolutionary, Food Enzyme Concept, a list of references cited in the book, has been appended to the text. It may, however, be mentioned that even at the time of writing the book Dr. Howell had accumulated over 700 scientific papers on this subject supporting his thesis, although only 400+ were actually cited in the book. This may give an idea to the interested reader as to how much material was available in this area even at that time. Since then, of course, many thousands of scientific papers have appeared on the subject matter of this book.

As an aid to a more thorough comprehension of the contents by the lay person, who is generally much more informed and aware of the close connection of nutrition with both physical and mental health than ever before, a glossary of scientific terms used in this book, is for the first time provided at the end of the subject matter. It is our sincerest wish and hope that the present format and additional information will not only lead to a greater understanding of the pioneer work of Dr. Howell, but will also help readers to make more informed decisions about their diet and its relationship with exuberant health and longevity!

PREFACE

In the year 1934, I prepared a short manuscript entitled, "*Are Food Enzymes Important in Digestion and Metabolism?*" and forwarded a copy to Professor H. C. Sherman, Columbia University, and another copy to Professor W. H. Howell, Johns Hopkins University, for comment and criticism. Since the concept was entirely new, it was deemed desirable to secure competent guidance. In the intervening years, I have received many valuable suggestions from specialists in the several sciences bearing on the subject. The present manuscript was written in the year 1939 and embodies some of the literature up to that time. Material not included in the present writing as well as data accumulated since 1939 will, it is hoped, be published subsequently.

Since the subject is new, it is not to be expected that the present effort can be anything more than a mere preamble to a more matured and extended compilation. I seek the help of those qualified to judge in pointing out to me by correspondence any errors of fact or logic that may appear in this work.

It is hoped that, because of the novelty of the food enzyme concept, the bold approach to the problem will be tolerated and recognized as necessary to stimulate the interest and development which the matter merits, and that minor errors of logic or fact may be excusable because of the urgency of formulating a panoramic presentation of the subject.

Edward Howell

Chicago, Illinois.
February 28,1946

Foreword to the 2014 Edition

ENZYMIZE OR DIE
(Copyright Rev. Viktoras Kulvinskas MS - HHEI, YS)

"To say that the body can easily digest and assimilate cooked foods may someday prove to be the most grievous oversight yet committed by science."
Enzyme Nutrition, Edward Howell M.D.

"Enzymes is the most promising word in research. Today, many researchers are convinced that virtually all disease can be traced to missing or faulty enzymes."
Today's Health Magazine, American Medical Association, 1962

"In the near future substantial developments in Pharmacology and Therapeutics can be expected of enzymes."
Pharmaceutical Chemistry And Biochemical Pharmacology -'Bible' of the Pharmacologists. Kirk and Othmer, 1994

"Biology will be to the 21st Century what physics and chemistry were to this century. The main area of interest will be the production of enzymes, or living catalysts, which will act in the same way as chemical catalysts."
Megatrends: Ten New Directions, John Naisbitt 1992

"If the organism is supplied with enzymes during the entire life-time, many diseases of advanced age would be reduced."
Enzymes in Health and Disease, Dr. Greenberg

"The nutrition of the future will be based upon the frequency of food and upon the contribution of that frequency to our physical, mental, emotional and spiritual energy-levels. Our ancestors consumed an enzyme-rich diet, and, without question, that diet is the nutritional basis of human creation. We have wandered from this simple-yet-profound biochemical truth. Enzymes are indubitably at the heart of physiological healing; and they also benefit brain-waves, thereby stabilizing and enhancing the emotions."

Dr. Brian Clement - Director of 'The Hippocrates Health Institute'

INTRODUCTION
PERSONAL JOURNEY WITH ENZYMES

Over 50 years ago, I was ignorant of enzymes. As a matter of fact, the word was not even part of the masses' nor my vocabulary. After I left a very exciting career in the computer industry, brought about by stress and abusive lifestyle habits, I reached out to what was then an underground community of natural healers.

I soon observed the healing results, not only of my own personal challenges, too many of which to mention, but also of the clients at Ann Wigmore's Rising Sun Christianity (which later became The Hippocrates Health Institute). I became fascinated by the exceptional recovery rates I observed in asthma, diabetes, paralysis, cardiovascular degeneration as well as cancer when the clients consumed a strictly raw food diet with a high intake of wheatgrass juice and sprouts. As I read much of the literature in the alternative health care industry, especially the works of Dr. Edmond Szekely and other health professionals, it became clear to me that the healing was facilitated by the re-introduction of food with very high enzyme content. I, therefore, became much more diligent in seeking out any studies of the therapeutic use of enzymes within the medical community.

What really brought all of my research and wisdom together in the most cutting edge synthesis of the theoretical foundation for enzymatic therapies was the work of Dr. Edward Howell. While doing research for over five years at Harvard Medical Library, I had the good fortune of discovering some of his abandoned manuscripts. In 1939 he had published a paper, Food Enzymes for the Effects on Digestion and Metabolism.

Dr. Howell had submitted his work to the top universities and medical doctors of his day in an attempt to propagate the concept that enzymes are, and will someday be discovered to be, an essential dietary nutrient. He concluded that a grave shift had been made in history when cooking was introduced. After reading his work, I was compelled to track him down. It took me several years to do so, and when I finally did he humbly agreed to allow me to publish his manuscripts and co-author this book, "Food Enzymes for Health and Longevity". I printed 10,000 copies at my own expense and initiated the circulation with a passion.

Upon its initial release into the public, the book was written using scientific language and unfortunately, at that time, enzymes were relatively new in the world of science. Thus, the book was not read by many and therefore did not become popular. However, while working at the Hippocrates Health Institute over the years that followed, I was eventually able to edit the text and make it more reader friendly and understandable.

I also had the opportunity to be trained by Dr. Howell in the production and formulation of enzymatic supplements. He had only one product at that time, which was a very low potency mixture of microbiologically created enzymes. I became a consultant and sales agent for his company along with a business partner. We took the manufacturing first to the direct sales markets and then to retail stores. Over time, the enzymes were made more potent, creating faster results, not only as digestive enzymes but also as systemic enzymes influencing therapeutically the function of the immune system and overflowing into the numerous metabolic processes of the body. Over time, my partner, Lee A. Wolfman, and I pioneered the development of systems of products that enabled us to address any condition through a series of specially designed enzyme, herbal and nutraceutical products. The company went from six employees to over 120 and, at its peak, was doing over 70 million dollars a year in business directly from the products that we had developed.

I have continued throughout the years that followed, right up into the now, being involved in the most revolutionary and pioneering work with enzymes. This exploration continues to be a significant piece of my personal history and contribution.

WHAT ARE ENZYMES?

Enzymes have a very ancient, longstanding history and are found in the culinary arts of most all cultures. Enzymes are created by the microbial cultures found within fermented foods. In the East there are fermentations of soy and other seeds by way of miso, tamari, tempeh and kimchi. In the West there are ferments such as yogurt, beer, wine and sauerkraut as well as other microbial concoctions. Of further note is the fact that recent studies demonstrate that populations who consume some form of fermented foods on a daily basis are noted to live longer as well as have lower rates of disease and infant mortality.

The root word "enzyme" comes from the Greek word "énzymo" which means "to ferment" or "to cause a change."

Enzymes are large biological molecules responsible for the thousands of metabolic processes that sustain life. They are highly selective catalysts, greatly accelerating both the rate and specificity of metabolic reactions, from the digestion of food to the synthesis of DNA. Most enzymes are proteins, although some catalytic RNA molecules have been identified.

WIKIPEDIA

Enzymes are the foundation for all cell regeneration. They play a key role in the transformation of undigested food into the nutrients that are absorbed on the cellular level. With proper nutrition, we have the energy to participate in the dance we call life.

An enzyme is a specialized protein structure that carries with it an energetic charge that sparks the symphony of life. Life is a divine electromagnetic orchestration of a galaxy of nutrients or micro-galactic systems of predominantly enzymes, which are the only nutrients in your body that are capable of doing any work. Either in breaking down complicated food to produce basic biological and useful substances or in the assembly of amino acids and other nutraceuticals which facilitate metabolism and all biological processes of life.

Enzymes speed up chemical reactions that normally take place very slowly or not at all. It is the energy behind the protein structure that makes enzymes different from other protein-based substances. However, when exposed to temperatures higher than 120° Fahrenheit, enzymes lose their ability to do biological work within the body and function more like proteins.

THE HEALTH CRISIS DUE
TO FOOD ENZYME DESTRUCTION

In the wilderness, among the animals there is neither illness such as acute colds and flues nor chronic conditions such as cancer. In the jungles of ongoing stress of who is going to be eating whom, it is far more intense than what we experience in our cement jungles of modern civilization. There is a reason why the wild animals are healthy, why gorillas can outdo in strength anybody trained in a modern gym or why the antelope can break the two-minute mile without pre-Olympic training. Essentially, optimal functioning comes down to living on alkalizing, enzymatic nutrition that is high in greens and appropriate to metabolic body type. A gorilla has a digestive and anatomical system similar to humans and it thrives on greens. The strongest and fastest animals are green eaters.

Through enzyme rich and living nutrition we embrace the process and creation of life. In contrast, from the consumption of enzyme-less, processed, cooked, and non-organic food we welcome "disease" and death.

In "Today's Health" (September 1960), published by the American Medical Association, Dr. Ratcliff states "many research men believe that the aging process is the result of the slowing down and disorganization of enzyme activity. Might it eventually be possible to restore youthful patterns of activity by supplying those enzymes that are deficient." Ratcliff goes on to say, "researchers are convinced that virtually all disease can be traced to missing or faulty enzymes. To date, an estimated forty-four diseases have been related to enzyme disturbances."

It is clear that the stress of eating cooked food compromises our digestive system, immune functions and metabolism. The following statistics indicate that the number one cause of absenteeism from work, visits to doctors, hospitalization, surgery, chronic diseases and death is due to poor digestion, which is created daily at every enzymeless meal.

Despite the fact that western medicine offers exceptional science, care, and treatment of trauma and accidents as well as improves the quality of life, it has failed to address the causes of degenerative diseases and has relied on methods that are very ineffective. Fortunately, a major trend in medicine presently is a shift towards non-invasive therapies that have shown to be very effective by organizations such as PCM.org, Integrated Medicine, Holistic Medical Association, Alternative Medical Association, as well as the evolving Lifestyle Medicine. All of these are offering great hope for the future.

Never the less, currently the high cost of enzyme deficiency in dollars, suffering and death is as follows:

- Over 700,000 Americans die each year at the hands of government-sanctioned medicine, while the FDA and other government agencies pretend to protect the public by harassing those who offer safe alternatives. In addition, the number of unnecessary medical and surgical procedures performed annually is 7.5 million per year and the number of people exposed to unnecessary hospitalization annually is 8.9 million per year.

- The stunning statistic that the total number of deaths caused by conventional medicine is an astounding 783,936 per year indicates that the American medical system is the leading cause of death and injury in the US.

- It is evident that the foundational cause of all sickness and "dis-ease' in the country is related to digestion. Statistics from the National Institutes of Health and the U.S. Department of Health and Human Services reveal that 60 to 70 million people are affected by all digestive diseases.

- In 2004, there were an estimated 72 million ambulatory care visits with a first-listed diagnosis of a digestive disease and more than 104 million visits with an all-listed diagnoses, which equated to a rate of 35,684 visits per 100,000 U.S. population. In other words, for every 100 U.S. residents, there were 35 ambulatory care visits at which a digestive disease diagnosis was noted.

- The largest individual disease contributions to the increase were made by gastro esophageal reflux disease (GERD), with an increase over this period of 376 per 100,000 population; viral hepatitis C, with 79 per 100,000; chronic constipation, with 62 per 100,000; intestinal infections, with 41 per 100,000; and pancreatitis, with 23 per 100,000.

- The total indirect cost of digestive diseases in the United States in 2004 was estimated at $44 billion. Almost three-quarters of these costs were due to mortality, and one-fourth was from work loss due to medical care or illness. Liver disease, colorectal cancer, and pancreatic cancer resulted in the greatest indirect costs.

- The total estimated cost of digestive diseases, including direct and indirect, in the United States in 2004 was $141.8 billion. Direct costs accounted for 69 percent of the total. The majority of costs (88 percent of direct and 92 percent of indirect) were assigned to specific digestive diseases. In total cost, the most costly diseases were liver disease ($13.1 billion), GERD ($12.6 billion), colorectal cancer ($9.5 billion), gallstones ($6.2 billion), and AWH ($6.1 billion).

(http://digestive.niddk.nih.gov/statistics/Digestive_Disease_Stats_508.pdf)

The above numbers and statistics are quite staggering especially when it's clear that including daily enzymes through either a living/uncooked diet and/or digestive enzyme supplementation would alleviate the vast majority of health issues that plague modern society.

An historical occurrence that clearly evidences the impact and effect of enzymes has been observed in the changes that took place in the Eskimo population. When their diet of animal protein was in an enzymatically rich state, eaten raw and or fermented, most lived into their 90's experiencing total health with a full set of teeth and a full head of hair. However, when the exploring missionaries and pioneers introduced cooked food to the Eskimos, within just one generation, those who adopted the cooked methods experienced a 50% drop in longevity, dying of cancer, acidosis and cardiovascular diseases as would be expected.

Thus, we see the destruction from cooking of lipase and protease leads to the eventual development of cancer, heart attacks and a radical reduction of longevity. I do not advocate the raw Eskimo diet of course, since even though it is enzymatically active it eventually leads to the development of acidosis. Furthermore, scientific and humanitarian reasoning show that a plant-based diet, which is cruelty free, is not only adequate but also sustainable for all life.

Dr. Dick Couey, Professor of Physiology and Nutrition at Baylor University in Texas stated, "I will never eat another meal without taking a plant enzyme supplement. My body doesn't deserve such poor treatment."

AMYLASE, LIPASE, AND PROTEASE

The three categories of digestive enzymes are amylase, lipase and protease. The deficiency of any one of these diminishes the quality of life eventually leading to acute symptoms such as colds, flues or aches followed by chronic illness such as cancer, heart conditions and other degenerative diseases. Numerous studies indicate that we have a crisis of deficiencies of these three enzyme groups. Insufficient enzymes plays a key role in all of our degenerative diseases, which in fact are essentially conditions and symptoms associated with incompletely metabolized starch, fat and/or protein. The continuation of the decomposition of these incompletely digested foods by yeast, pathogenic microbes and a wide variety of parasites further accelerates the degeneration process.

Without adequate enzymes the immune system is compromised and the daily toxicity from the environmental and other stresses ends up accumulating within the human organism. Dr. James B. Sumner, a 1946 Nobel Prize recipient and Professor of Biochemistry at Cornell University, wrote in his book, "The Secret of Life – Enzymes", that the "getting old feeling" after forty is due to depleted enzyme reserves, with amylase levels at almost zero. Young cells contain a hundred times more enzymes than old cells. Old cells are filled with metabolic waste and toxins. When we have indigestion from starch it quickly turns to acid, creating that acidic, burning situation. As a result, many people require Rolaids, Tums or some other acid reflux drug. This condition can easily be remedied with digestive enzymes that include a strong amylase foundation. Thus, we see that a deficiency of amylase starch digesting enzyme is one of the leading causes of the full range of symptoms of acidosis, which eventually ends up as acid crystal precipitants throughout the system agitating the neurological functioning and creating the acute and chronic pain that is plaguing modern man.

Dr. Guyton, of Tufts Medical School, states that obesity is strongly due to an insufficient level of lipase, the fat-splitting enzyme. Inadequate levels of protease and lipase lay the foundation for all major degenerative diseases and weight gain. During my long-term commitment with Dick Gregory's Morbid Obesity Research Center, I observed that when I added a supplement of high lipase to the program it had a significant impact. With these extremely overweight clients, we witnessed that with the additional enzymes, the daily weight loss went from an original average of half a pound a day to over a pound, and in some cases as high as two pounds per day.

We have a pandemic of overweight and morbid obesity that is affecting over 60% of our population, primarily due to lipase deficiency. It is evident that this tragic statistic can be significantly lowered by enzyme supplementation. Of course, for the most effective outcomes, various lifestyle habits are also in need of improvement, especially exercise and a healthy positive attitude.

ENZYMES, HEALTH, AND HEALING
Beginning in the 1930's and spanning over two decades, Professor Edmond Szekely treated over 250,000 individuals successfully with early versions of "Living Enzymatic Food Therapy" at Rancho

La Puerta in Tecate, Baja California, Mexico. The professor truly gave a rebirth to what is referred to as the "Essene Biogenic Way of Life" and thereby to alternative therapies, as well as set the pace for a new level of healing and regeneration.

Professor Szekely's work was based on the Essene Dead Sea Scrolls and The Essene Gospel of Peace Volume One in which the historian Josephus records the accounts from over 2,000 years ago of the Essene group. This community, of over 4000 people, was noted for exceptional longevity, 400% longer than the rest of the Mediterranean region as well as being known for their happy, healthy and holy dispositions. Their biogenic nutrition was plant-based and included the consumption of high enzyme rich foods.

"For if you eat living food, the same will quicken you; if you kill your food, the dead food will kill you."

Jesus the Christ "The Essene Gospel of Peace", Dr. Edmond B. Szekely

As many of you may know, the modern evolution of plant-based therapies is the result of the pioneering work of Dr. Ann Wigmore and myself. We co-founded The Hippocrates Health Institute where our research was conducted. Our contribution has a long historic precedence despite the fact that we were working in complete isolation of the ongoing global healing therapies that were using raw, enzymatically-activated foods.

Over the last half century, I have had the opportunity to observe the success of the nutritional approach at Hippocrates Health Institute in solving the condition of cancer. Throughout the years we've become more holistic, improving our nutritional program, addressing emotional, mental and/or spiritual issues, as well as incorporating cardiovascular exercise with the most optimal supplementation available. The results continue to become more consistent with a more rapid and broader range of recovery.

Understanding the development of cancer and its reversal, by bringing the individual back to optimal wellness, had been a mystery that was revealed to me through the eyes of science, common sense, clinical experience and meditation.

According to Dr. Paul Zane Pilzer, in his book "The Wellness Revolution", a huge opportunity exists in helping the sick through the alternative care modalities. We are looking at radical expansion of the holistic treatment of all diseases that has as its key driving force of all successful treatment, the following: restoration of the enzymatic terrain, overcoming micronutrient malnutrition, subjecting one to detoxification, and immersing yourself into holistic lifestyles.

Dr. Max Wolfe, of Fordham University Department of Medicine and pioneering author of enzymology, showed a 95% recovery of all forms of cardiovascular disease, again with enzyme saturation.

"Indigestion due to greasy foods is common. [Plant-based] enzymes are helpful for weak digestion [common] in old age, or for digestive disturbances. Enzymes are helpful with large, rich meals or hard-to-digest food."

"Enzyme Therapy", Max Wolfe M.D.

The following discussion will explore and illustrate how protease enzymes play a key role in the recovery from all forms of cancer and heart diseases.

ENZYMES, PROTEINS, AND COOKED FOOD

On May 23, 2002 The New York Times Science Section released a lengthy report based on many clinical studies that revealed the fact that 100% of Americans on the S.A.D. (Standard American Diet) are saturated with incompletely metabolized protein, often referred to as "misfolded protein". The article went on to state that circulatory protein creates an inflammatory condition which keeps the immune system actively engaged 24 hours a day in detoxifying the body from this excess of protein waste. The many clinical studies in this article concluded that most likely all degenerative diseases including Alzheimer's, asthma, emphysema, Parkinson's, cardiovascular, and MS are caused by this phenomena.

Where do these misfolded proteins come from? Scientific research evidences that the greatest source of misfolded proteins are the ones that have been exposed to radiation, cooking and other forms of processing that change them into forms that our digestive enzymes are unable to convert into amino acids. Studies conducted by the USDA show that a 4 to 30 times increase of insoluble, indigestible protein fragments occurs under the duress of cooking at 400 degrees Fahrenheit, a common setting in baking and frying temperatures. Furthermore, in the Nutritional Review it showed that in dry heating, as in microwave ovens, grilling and other similar devices found at many restaurants, the essential amino acid of lysine is totally disorganized and fails to be digested by the protease enzymes. Other studies show that protein cooked with sugars and simple carbs leads to a loss of 50-84% of the essential amino acids. There are many other studies that demonstrate the impact of heat treatment, specific to the production of disorganized and misfolded proteins under the duress of cooking. As an overall statement on the subject, Dr. Spengler of the Institute of Traumatology showed that there is an inverse relationship between longevity and the consumption of heat-treated protein: the more you consume the shorter is your lifespan (see Survival in the 21st Century, page 46).

Dr. John Gainer showed that even a slight increase in heat-treated dietary protein "reduces oxygen transport by as much as 60% even though the amount of incompletely metabolized protein in the fluid would be considered within the normal range for human blood." Thus, a diet with a high volume of heat-treated protein can reduce the oxygen-carrying capacity of the blood thereby producing oxygen starvation, which eventually leads to asphyxiation. Clearly, heat-treated proteins create a major stress that is challenging your life process, since all metabolic and biological processes are dependent upon oxygen.

Nobel Prize recipient, Dr. Alexis Carrel, in his book "Man, The Unknown" states that "the human body in every form of stress, adapts itself by innovating systems that will allow the body to live through stressful experiences, though at the expense of longevity and vitality". Thus, the ingestion of dead, stressed, enzyme-less, cooked protein triggers inherent mechanisms in the body that are totally natural and are in fact activated to save your life. These mechanisms are otherwise known as cancer and cardiovascular disease.

ENZYMES, CANCER, AND CARDIOVASCULAR DISEASE

Dr. Ernst Froyd discovered that an individual that has been diagnosed with cancer by an oncologist can also go to a cardiologist and most often will also find some form of cardiovascular degeneration in need of treatment. Both conditions seem to co-exist with each other because both are assisting simultaneously in the management of heat-treated protein.

First, let's take a look at the cancer mechanism. There are approximately ten trillion chemical reactions going on in your body every second, all of which are oxygen-related. Life would cease to exist without adequate oxygen. Noble Prize Winner, Dr. Otto Warburger, in 1936 showed the fundamental cause of cancer. His research took normal reproductive cells and placed them in a petri dish with an optimal nutrient solution and placed it in an isolated, glass dome. When he reduced the normal oxygen level of the cells by 35%, within 48 hours the weaker cells died out while those remaining mutated into cancer cells. There is evidence to indicate that the production of these cancer cells serves an important function.

The cancer mechanism appears to be an innovative method of the human body to adapt itself to the stresses associated with heat-treated protein, the various toxins of society, and the breakdown of one's own body tissue. Each of the above leads to an exaggerated volume of incompletely metabolized cellular protein debris, which interferes with critical oxygen transport and its absorption. Cancer cells attempt to clean up the circulatory system in an effort to allow the life process to continue, which are dependent on oxygen.

University of Wisconsin discovered that cancer cells absorb protein 20 times faster than normal reproductive cells, which do a good job of absorbing amino acids but a poor job in absorbing undigested protein. Thus, we see how the cancer cells gather the circulatory protein allowing normal oxygen transport to go on.

Dr. Albert Lorincz, at The University of Chicago, starved cancer cells into submission by withholding protein elements essential to their development. The demand of cancer cells for protein is 1.3 to 11 times the level necessary for normal tissue. That's a profound discovery for sure.

Finally, Drs. Lepage and Midler confirmed the cancer nitrogen trap (or protein dumps) "vacuum cleaner" hypothesis. In a review of studies related to the nutrition of tumors they showed that over-nutrition, an excess intake of proteins and fats, has a definite effect on the development of cancer.

In essence, cancer is a life-saving strategy. If the body did not create it one would die rapidly due to asphyxiation.

CANCER IS A NATURAL RESPONSE OF THE IMMUNE SYSTEM

Cancer cells are similar to white blood cells in that both are part of the immune system and serve a very important function. Dr. Michael Williams, immunologist and professor of medicine at

Northwestern University, states that there are tens of thousands of cancerous cells floating around in our bodies at all times. This is in agreement with the position taken by most oncologists.

Cancer cells remove the incompletely metabolized proteins from the body. Accordingly, the cancer cell count is directly related to the level of oxygen depletion caused by incomplete metabolized proteins as well as anemic conditions. In essence, the less oxygen the more cancer cells.

The purpose of the white blood cells is to identify and remove microbial, pathogenic, viral and environmental metabolic waste/ toxins from the blood system. The white blood cell count goes up by over 300 % after every enzymeless meal. The white blood cells are created to gather enzymes from the metabolic enzyme pool, so that the cooked food can be digested with the help of these new enzymes. As the enzyme levels within the body diminish due to aging or poor lifestyle habits the amount of white blood cells created to assist in the harvesting of enzymes continues to increase.

Normally, in a healthy individual, within a few hours after a cooked meal the white blood cell count goes back to normal. However, if the individual continues to snack throughout the day as well as be exposed to environmental pollutants, the body is in a continuous inflammatory state and the white blood cell count continues to increase. Eventually the volume of the increased count interferes with the transport of nutrients as well as the removal of waste products and detoxification, thereby leading to the wasting away disease of acute and chronic leukemia.

Just as exaggerated volumes of white blood cells create a disease called leukemia, so is it that exaggerated volumes of cancer cells create other forms of cancer. As volume of the cancer sacks of excess protein increases year by year, eventually it begins to interfere with ones' normal biological processes. Organs are displaced and getting in the way of function, circulation and elimination creating such conditions as colon cancer and the other various diagnosis of chronic cancer.

Initially, white blood and cancer cells serve the important function of removing the stress of blood pollutants and extending life rather than allowing the destruction that can be caused by these toxins. Just as white blood cells are natural and normal in supporting the life process, so too are the cancer cells. It's all a matter of the numbers, too many of either one interferes with the balance and thereby the biological process of life.

The body will always borrow enzymes from different organs for digestive support if one is not eating living foods or taking enzyme supplements. Evidence of this is greatly shown by the activity of the white blood cells, which travel around the body in response to a variety of digestive disorders. This medical phenomenon is called "post-meal leukocytosis" and has been studied extensively by Dr. Paul Kouchakoff. As stated above, he shows that there is a 300-500% increase in white blood cells after the cooked meals whereas there is no increase in white blood cell count when the meal is enzymatically active. As we know, the purpose of white blood cells is to deal with inflammatory conditions.

ENZYME THERAPY FOR CANCER

The saturation of the body with enzymes has been shown in a variety of studies to have many successful reversals of cancer.

In the beginning of the century, John Beard's incredible book, "Enzyme Therapy for Cancer and Its Scientific Basis", truly set a new scientific standard in the field of enzymology. He states that every form of cancer is preceded by pancreatic insufficiency and the breakdown of its ability to supply adequate enzymes.

Similar wisdom is also quoted in Dr. Max Gerson's book, "A Cancer Therapy: Results of Fifty Cases and the Cure of Advanced Cancer by Enzymatic Diet Therapy." His groundbreaking research using alkalizing, enzymatic nutrition by way of carrot and green vegetable juices proved to have a high rate of healing recovery from cancer. Gerson states that when enzyme levels diminish due to the eating of enzyme-less foods the body has to harvest enzymes from the metabolic pool as well as compromise the enzyme usage by the immune system. If food is not digested properly then the proteins rot, creating over 35 organic, slow acting acids. We also know that these incompletely metabolized proteins get through the gut barrier and tremendously interfere with oxygen transport. Likewise, the fats that turn rancid also get across that barrier causing blood cells to clot.

Unfortunately, the enzymeless therapies for cancer often show themselves to be more lethal than helpful. According to cancer researcher Dr. Hardin B. Jones, "Those who fail to get any kind of treatment for cancer, outlive those who go the cut, burn and/or chemical route." His research shows that those who get modern medical treatment barely live three years, while those who refuse treatment live an average of 12.5 years.

There are many pioneering works that are using enzymes alone as a way of favorably impacting the reversal of the cancer condition. Enzyme therapy without medical intervention and/or without removing the seminal cause of the cancer has proven to be effective in numerous cases.

Dr. Ottokar Rokitansky believes enzyme treatment is effective in conjunction with surgery and chemotherapy because: cancer cells are more sensitive to proteolytic enzymes than normal body cells; enzymes dissolve the fibrin coating on the cancer cells, allowing the body's defenses to function better, and; enzymes can diminish the stickiness of the cancer cell, preventing the formation of metastases.

Dr. A.E. Leskovar reported that supplementation with enzymes increases the macrophages by 700% and natural killer cells by 1,300% in a short time. Dr. Michael Williams states that when "enzyme levels are adequate," immune system scavenger cells called macrophages destroy abnormal cells, keeping their numbers in check. Dr. Chin Po Kim successfully treated all forms of cancer with enzymes, producing a 79% recovery rate in a double blind study that included a five-year follow up. No other lifestyle changes were initiated other than orally administered enzymes.

The following study showed that radically reducing the heat-treated protein in the diet led to reducing the need of enzymes for digestion thereby creating a surplus of enzymes to be used for immune function and recovery from leukemia. Lancet and Polish Medical Journal report Dr. Kalikowski's results where a low protein diet was used in conjunction with high alkaline solutions to cure leukemia: "favorable effects in 10 out of 13 children with leukemia and a strikingly fast disappearance of blast cells in bone marrow was noted compared to controls." Of further note is that one of the reasons given for lack of complete success was that they had not yet devised an optimal diet.

By reducing the protein intake, the amount of enzymes needed to process the protein is reduced, which has a favorable effect on the incidence of cancer. Dr. Saxton showed in a study that normal feeding of a leukemia susceptible strain of mice produced a 6.5 times higher incidence of leukemia than in mice kept on a strict diet. Also noted was that the length of life of these mice was considerably prolonged by underfeeding.

Whether with or without medical intervention, it seems clear that enzymes jump-start the immune function thus creating a radical healing of cancer.

ENZYMES AS TREATMENT AND PREVENTION OF CANCER
All the above-mentioned therapies have done nothing to removing the cause of the cancer; the partial solution initiated by enzyme saturation does not address the initial and extensive pollution/

toxemia introduced by the heat-treated proteins, which bring about other health crises such as acidosis eventually leading to termination of life.

At The Hippocrates Health Institute, most individual's transition from eating high levels of heat-treated proteins to a diet that is made up of organic, non-GMO greens and enzymatically pre-digested foods, which are alkalizing to the body. At Hippocrates they use not only the most advanced enzyme supplement saturation of their cancer clients but also address and remove the accumulated causes for the initiation of the cancer mechanism within the human body. This is accomplished by avoiding not only heat-treated proteins but also all forms of fruit and sugar concentrates, which in fact provide energy for the cancer cells. Essentially, ensuring that the individuals have their biomarkers reset namely by re-alkalizing, re-enzymizing, re-oxygenating, re-bacterizing and re-mineralizing accomplish the success experienced at Hippocrates. Not only does this lead to overall rejuvenation, but also to a more youthful life as long as one maintains at least an 80% living foods and 20% cooked (with enzymatic supplementation) organic, whole food program. Accordingly, Hippocrates has the highest rate of recovery in all of the cancer treatment industry.

At present, the Hippocrates Program is currently being researched in conjunction with The University of California School of Medicine. While medical doctors consider Stage 4 breast cancer incurable, it is consistently reversed to recovery within a five-month period through the Hippocrates holistic approach. These results are undoubtedly of great interest and inspiration to many.

CARDIOVASCULAR HEALTH
AND ENZYME DEFICIENCY

My success with the German translated version of my book, "Survival in the 21st Century" resulted in me receiving a letter from a German medical student with a complete translation of the following Wendt study. This research showed that surplus protein ends up being stored within the 60,000 miles of blood vessels, thus working in parallel and simultaneously with cancer in cooperation as to the management of the toxic circulation of incompletely metabolized protein. One might say that as the cancer cells make an effort to vacuum up the protein, the cardiovascular system attempts to sweep it into the basement membrane of the blood vessels.

For 30 years the Wendts, a family of research physicians, developed evidence 'o show that those who ingest too much (animal) protein ac.ually develop a generalized Protein Storage Disease. The Wendts showed, through the use of Electron Microscope Photography, that excess protein results in the clogging of the Basement Cell Membranes (BCMs). BCMs are those through which nutrients and oxygen are filtered into the cells from the capillaries and through which the waste products of the cells are filtered out into the blood to be eliminated.

Eventually the BCMs becomes so clogged that nutrients and oxygen are not able to pass into the cells and the waste products cannot be eliminated. The results are decreased oxygen in the cell and subsequent cellular malnutrition. In the Wendts' observations, the (animal) protein builds up in such a way that it contributes to cancer, hypertension, atherosclerosis, cardiovascular (heart) disease, and adult-onset TYPE 2 diabetes.

As the lymphatic and cardiovascular system piles up with muco-phlegm there are malignancies that end up storing all that extra protein with a less than optimal effect and the life process becomes threatening. In conclusion, it appears that the human body is undoubtedly best served by implementing a program of enzyme therapy.

WHOLE FOOD ENZYMATIC
NUTRITION FOR WELLNESS
The nutritional value of food can no longer be simply calculated

by calories, proteins, fats and carbohydrates because none of these components can be properly assimilated without their active enzymes. Enzymes are now being understood to be an associated member of food contents along with vitamins and minerals.

It's important to keep in mind that minerals play a vital role in the digestion and assimilation of essential nutrients needed for the proper functioning of the body. It is estimated that 99% of Americans are deficient in one or more essential minerals (US Government Document No. 264). Minerals are the catalysts for the enzyme systems. Enzymes systems make life possible. The minerals are essential to enzyme systems either because they are part of the enzyme itself, or they act as co-factors, which enable the enzymes to work properly. We now understand that minerals in excess can put stress on bodily functions, and it is therefore advisable that the most effective way to take in minerals is from whole foods, such as the fresh water algae, sea vegetables and land grasses.

As one's enzyme reserves continue to diminish, more and more of the incompletely metabolized food not only creates rot and putrefaction along the gastro intestinal tract but can also instigate leaky gut syndrome and ulcerations. These kind of conditions lead to the internal absorption of incompletely metabolized protein, starch and fat. This in turn, creates a major interference with the normal metabolic processes, especially the transport of oxygen to the body, as well as the effective detoxification of the blood by liver, kidney and lung activity.

ENZYME-RICH NUTRITION
Continued research in enzyme therapeutics concludes that the model of enzymatically rich and alkaline green nutrition combined with enzymatic supplementation radically accelerates any kind of recovery process.

A classic book, "Enzymes, The Fountain of Life" by MD's Lopez,

Williams and Miehlke reinvigorated the standard of enzyme wisdom. This work has since been continued by others like Dr. Nicholas Gonzalez in his books such as his most recent, "What Went Wrong: The Truth Behind the Clinical Trial of the Enzyme Treatment of Cancer".

At the University of Southern California, Dr. Hunt conducted extremely interesting studies involving both those who consumed food that lacked enzymes and those who consumed food that was rich in enzymes. The electromagnetic field of the bodies of those who consumed enzymeless food or "void nutrition" diminished. By contrast, the electromagnetic energy of those who consumed raw vegetarian food increased dramatically.

F.J. Sweeney studied the injuries of 100 professional and college athletes who were taking enzymes supplements daily. He obtained marked results in 87% of the athletes and moderate results in 10% of the cases, particularly in the reduction of edema, associated pain and return of full activity of the injured area. ("Treatment of Athletic Injuries with an Oral Proteolytic Enzyme", Medical Times, 1963).

That said, not all enzymes are created equal...

NOT ALL ENZYMES
ARE CREATED EQUAL

Many enzymes taken to aid digestion such as pepsin, trypsin, and pancreatin, are derived from animal sources. They have a very narrow window of viability in terms of pH conditions, working in either just the small intestine or the stomach. When the pH level gets either too high or too low, these enzymes are deactivated. Consequently, when people take these types of enzymes, they do not receive the expected nutritional assistance required. In the final analysis, the research shows that for the most part, animal enzymes will ultimately do more harm than good. In contrast, naturally derived non-animal enzymes have a much wider range of pH adaptability, working throughout the digestive system and thereby not requiring enteric coating.

Clearly, when seeking out any kind of enzyme supplementation it is always best to do your research and really know your source, including the methods used to create the product. When choosing a plant-based enzyme it is important to make sure that the description of the digestive components is not in units of weight, such as milligrams, but rather units of activity. For example, the total protease levels should be at least 50,000 HUTs, the amylases at least 10,000 units of activity, and the lipase at least 500 HUTs. All of the above activity should be contained within a complex diversity of enzyme components and co-factors. The largest component in your body after water is protein, hence it is best to utilize the most diversified protease complex with an adjunct of nutraceutical extracts such as AstraGin®, which will lead to maximizing your cellular absorption of the total digested protein. The development of this extract in 2014 is one of the greatest breakthroughs in enzymology with respect to enzymatic action and the absorption of nutrients.

RECENT RESEARCH CONFIRMS THE
POWER OF A UNIQUE ENZYME COMBINATION.

In 2014, Enzymology Research Center, Inc. released a landmark study that utilized AstraXymeTM, a unique combination of proteolytic enzymes and trace minerals along with extracts of Astragalus membranaceus and Panax notoginseng (AstraGin®). The study was divided into two parts. The first half of the study showed a 90% - 96% breakdown of a protein (bovine hemoglobin, the standard used in protein digestion studies) into peptides and amino acids in pH ranges from 4.0 – 10.0 that are found in the human digestive tract. The second half of the study confirmed that 40% more peptides and amino acids were absorbed into the intestinal cells while also increasing the absorption rates by over 30%.

The two findings have very important implications with regards to digestion, immune function, and overall health. Protein in foods and supplements cannot be utilized by the human body unless they are broken down into smaller peptides or amino acids. Undigested protein or protein that is not completely broken down can lead to a number of serious health issues. This study shows that taking plant-based proteolytic enzymes with a unique trace mineral blend "digested" close to 100% of the protein.

The second equally important benefit is the improvement in the absorption function so more peptides and amino acids are taken in and retained in the body to nourish its trillions of cells. A growing body of scientific research indicates that the absorption function in the general population is in decline due to a combination of the modern diet, an increase in the use of medication, and elevated stress levels. Another contributing factor is the demographics of the rapidly aging population of "baby boomers" who, by the very nature of their "senior status", have severely compromised digestive function. This reality is evidenced by the increasing sales of digestive-related over the counter drugs. Conditions such as bloating, constipation, diarrhea, indigestion,

IBD, Crohn's disease, and "Leaky Gut Syndrome" (Excessive Intestinal Permeability) are on the rise. The AstraGin®1 complex has been shown in over a dozen studies to increase the absorption of many amino acids, certain vitamins, as well as other important human nutrients. Additionally, AstraGin® has been shown in multiple In vivo studies to increase the absorption of cationic amino acids (e.g. arginine, lysine, and histidine) in normal rats and even in rats whose intestinal walls were damaged. More importantly, AstraGin® actually repaired the damaged intestinal wall, which is where most nutrients are absorbed, leading to the restoration and improvement of the absorption function.

AstraXymeTM is the first and only digestive health supplement that addresses the importance of both the "digestion" (bioavailability) and the "absorption" functions. The old saying, "you are what you eat", which has more recently been updated in some circles to be a bit more accurate by stating, "you are what you digest," can now find its ultimate evolution in the following form: "you are what you eat, what you digest and what you absorb."

1. AstraGin® is a registered trademark of NuLiv Science USA, Inc. AstraXyme™ is a trademark of Enzymology Research Center, Inc. For more details please see Appendix II.

The human body and all living systems are, by Natural Law, self-sustaining, self-healing and self-regenerating. Perhaps it is time to shift our attention away from the degeneration process and refocus it on the regeneration process. That being said, enzymes will no doubt prove, once again, to be the key component of regeneration on the cellular level. When this process of cellular regeneration is aggregated at the level of the organism we call this rejuvenation, or as I prefer to call it, Youthing™. For more on Youthing™ see www.youthing.com.

CONCLUDING THOUGHTS

In summary, whether you incorporate more enzymes into your life by eating raw foods, purchasing enzyme supplements, or growing enzymes on your own remember the principles outlined above. You can be your own doctor, create your own enzymes and heal yourself inexpensively, simply and joyfully at home. All the enzymatically-rich food that you need can be produced organically through sprouting and growing micro-

greens cultivated either with or without soil. Additionally, one can learn to produce their own fermented products such as seed cheeses, kimchi, and sauerkraut.

Of course, one must always keep in mind that there are other activities that also contribute tremendously to a full spectrum healing and vibrant recovery from any health challenge/ opportunity. Some important elements to include in any program of prevention or healing are meditation, exercise, adequate rest, proper hydration, attitude modification, as well as mental and environmental upgrades through love and connection with others.

We are enzymatically changing our planet through laughter, simplicity, honor and action. When we tend to our inner garden we are then more able to share our love and our vibrant energy for life with others. What else is there? We are entering a new era of humanity where billions of people will operate within a singular union with what we call Mother Gaia. This is a paradigm shift to complete cooperation instead of competition. This level of collaboration is analogous to one's trillions of cells cooperating and co-creating the healthy body and consciousness that is you. May we continue to deepen our knowing of this experience both within our own selves and in connection with others.

PEACE REIGNS,
Rev. Viktoras Kulvinskas, MS.

CONTENTS

INTRODUCTION

As an author, researcher and observer in the raw food diet for therapy and maintenance for the past fifteen years, I am overwhelmed to discover Dr. Howell's book through the National Enzyme Co. I have been searching for and experimenting with exogenous (outside) digestive enzymes for many years in an attempt to allow folks to supplement their cooked food transition (or maintenance) diet. The best book on exogenous enzymes, which I discovered was the work of Dr. Howell, *"The Status of Food Enzymes in Digestion and Metabolism"*. He found plant enzymes in capsules best for predigestion. I was amazed that this book was written in 1939 at a time when most doctors knew nothing about vitamins and minerals and very few had heard the word "enzyme".

A classic is a work that is timeless. Although forty years have passed since it was written, today the book is more relevant than it ever was. Its truths need to be applied by all students of health and nutrition. I feel that it is one of the most important books to be published in the field of scientific nutrition.

Dr. Howell goes beyond everyone else and creates a scientific model for the treatment of all diseases and the maintenance of perfect health that supersedes all other attempts at nutritional therapy. His approach is grounded in tradition (Genesis 1:29), the patterns of natural nutrition in animals, and sound cultural ecological dietary practices. Further, he is presenting one of the most heated, controversial and exciting debates in the history of dietary consideration - raw foods versus cooked. His story is highly readable, at times entertaining, giving full counterarguments. No region of importance is left uncovered. It can be read easily by the lay person, and inspire such a person to make dietary alterations, as well as expanding the science of nutrition such that diet will become the main tool for healing most of the existent physical and mental disorders. I believe that if we apply the enzyme rich raw food diet in therapy, and as a goal to be realized in the gradual dietary transition where each year one consumes larger quantities of raw food, then we will eliminate disease and increase each generation's longevity, and possibly even reach the spectacular ages of Methuselah and other Biblical patriarchs.

If pioneers of science were still being burned as in the past for proposing new interpretations which later become gospel truths, I would not give much for the life of Dr. Howell. "A new scientific truth does not triumph by convincing its opponents by making them see the light, but rather because its opponents eventually die and a new generation is familiar with it." Since Dr. Howell's book is already two generations old, we are finding greater receptivity among the scientific and lay communities as the opponents die off from their faulty dietary habits. A deep change in science will come about only when we have conscious, responsible scientists who see nature as a partner and bring wisdom to the layman so that they too apply nature's law to heal self and the planet.

Enzymes effect our existence. They have been applied in every phase of healing from arthritis, diabetes, heart disorders and cancer, as well as in agriculture, dairy and wine fermentation, and the biological transmutation of one element into another. Without enzymes, we develop problems.

The United States is ecologically in bad shape. The planet is polluted because the mind and spirit have lost contact with nature due to processed, devitalized foods which are clogging the bloodstream with poor nutrition thus attenuating the oxygen supply to the brain and all body parts. Bodies deficient in nutrients and overloaded with toxic waste are creating an epidemic in the United States where 65% of Americans are chronically ill and 20% of teenagers are suffering from premature aging.

What is so amazing is that although the universities and private research firms with budgets totaling in the billions of dollars have not managed to achieve a major breakthrough in the healing of the epidemic chronic disease, yet, nevertheless, a single man, forty years ago, could provide an answer to all human ailments as well as to aging. Dr. Howell comes to such a basic, yet controversial conclusion that many, if not all degenerative diseases that Americans suffer from, are doctored for and die from are chiefly caused by eating cooked foods and produce deficient in enzymes. His research is the first significant scientific attempt to show the importance of raw foods in human nutrition. His work basically shows that science made a great mistake when it endorsed cooked food eating, a mistake which has led to the development of one of the sickest nations in the world.

Today many researchers are catching up with and extending the pioneer work of Dr. Howell. There is a significant turn of events in research, for example in the study of cancer, where few highly respected researchers are relating the disease to enzyme deficiency which could be prevented and possibly reversed through live food dietary management. Some of these researchers are: Dr. Arthur Robinson, Linus Pauling Institute of Science and Medicine; Dr. Chiu Nan Lai, University of Texas System Cancer Center, M.D. Anderson Hospital and Tumor Institute; Dr. Max Gerson, author of "*Cancer: 51 Cases*"; Professor William Salter, Yale Medical School.

Already, during the first week of 1980, a cancer study by the National Cancer Institute approved the first clinical trial of laetrile and enzymes on humans in conjunction with a "special metabolic diet" (the terminology used to designate a diet of predominantly raw foods according to the explanation I received from the research project spokesman). Last year two health journals, "*Let's Live*" and "*Bestways*", which are among the journals with the largest circulation, strongly advocated a modified raw food diet.

The live food program that Dr. Ann Wigmore and myself developed at the Hippocrates Health Institute, Boston, has proven to be effective in the prevention and reversal of degenerative disease, besides providing a tasty and efficient maintenance diet. It is the diet most rich in enzymes. It is inexpensive, can be totally organic, and grown even in a city apartment.

Leukemia is a classic area for the study of this raw foods diet. Genetically predisposed individuals will develop leukemia on a poor quality diet. Raw food will help to alleviate the condition by eliminating the excess of leukocytes produced due to cooked food.

"'Leukocytosis' is the name that medical pathology gives to an excessive augment of white blood corpuscles in the blood. Donders discovered the phenomenon in 1846 and Virchow classified 'digestive leukocytosis' as 'normal' since everyone seemed to suffer from it. This was upset by Dr. Paul Kautchakoff, M.D., who showed that the cooking of food was the cause of leukocytosis. The white blood corpuscles prevent infection and intoxication of the blood. Kautchakoff found that he could divide his findings on leukocytosis in four distinct groups according to reaction in the blood: 1) raw food produced no augment in white blood cells of the blood; 2) common cooked food caused leukocytosis; 3) pressure cooked food caused greater leukocytosis than non-pressure cooked food; 4) manufactured foods such as wine, vinegar, white sugar, ham, etc. are the most offensive. Kautchakoff was no vegetarian yet his findings show that flesh would have to be eaten raw to avoid leukocytosis which would be unpalatable to humans, but prepared meat (cooked, smoked, salted, etc.) brought on the most violent reaction equivalent to the leukocytosis count manifest in poisoning."

Why this pathological condition exists after eating cooked food can be best explained by the fact that the cooked food is totally devoid of enzymes it has stored up in order to break down the food components into units small enough to enter the blood and lymph. The Leukocytes are rich in enzymes and are being transported to the stomach area to aid in the digestive process. They also carry on similar functions in the time of colds and other germ related diseases; in such cases they digest the foreign particles or protein based invading germs.

The condition of leukemia manifests in genetically predisposed individuals on a cooked and processed food diet. The body has been sensitized to overact in production of white blood enzyme rich cells when the pancreas is malfunctioning and supplying very few digestive enzymes. Furthermore, the condition is associated with higher amounts of uric acid and a weakened kidney. The white blood cells are being utilized to compensate, very ineffectively, for the mentioned deficiencies, by trying to digest - eat up - the foreign protein and excess uric acid. The cooked foods, according to Kautchakoff trigger off increased production of leukocytes, and Howell shows that they are acting as digestants.

Many successful therapies have been reported based on natural diets. Most researchers are finding leukemia to be the easiest of all cancers to correct. At Hippocrates Health Institute, I witnessed two cases of leukemia, one of ten years duration, heal on a raw food regimen in six weeks time. Also, *Lancet* and *Polish Medical Journal* report Dr. Kalikowski's studies where low protein diet was used, in conjunction with high alkaline solutions, to cure leukemia; "favorable effects in ten out of thirteen children with leukemia... a strikingly fast disappearance of blast cells in bone marrow was noted compared to controls." One of the reasons given for lack of complete success was that they had not yet devised an optimal diet.

At the Survival Foundation research farm I witnessed several astonishing cases of reversal of disease this past summer: a young man who was to be on insulin, according to the "best" authorities, for the rest of his life, gradually reduced from eighty units to none in two weeks; a woman with uterine cancer and low energy was relieved of all symptoms in two months; another woman, using up to twenty pills daily to control pain for over ten years, stopped use of all drugs in one day without further recurrence of headaches now for three months; a middle-aged leukemia patient after fifteen years of chemotherapy found a program that returned the white and red blood cell count to normal in six weeks. There are thousands of success stories like that. One point in common is reliance upon a high enzyme predigested live food diet consisting of sprouts, seed and vegetable ferments, and live juices from baby greens, fresh fruits and vegetables.

I have been working many years with such a diet for maintenance and therapy. The success of this program with degenerative diseases - including cancer and other "incurable" diseases - is overwhelming. I have not run into a single case where recovery was not possible provided the patient had not been destroyed irreversibly by surgery, chemotherapy, or radiation. Even in such cases encouraging results have been obtained.

Today many papers are being published by medical clinics and universities which have been influenced by our dietary studies. The work in the field of cancer with wheatgrass and raw food diet has been done by Dr. Arthur Robinson (Linus Pauling Institute) and Dr. Chiu Nan Lai (Anderson Hospital, Houston, Texas). In *Annals of Internal Medicine*, 1977, Dr. John Douglas, who used raw foods with high success in the treatment of diabetes, states, "My rationale is that since early man lived entirely on raw foods perhaps such a diet would be less stressful to the human system in general and less likely to produce diabetes than a cooked diet".

One of the most exciting recent developments in raw foods research is showing that raw inorganic produce are safer than cooked. Dr. William Newsome of Canada's Department of Health and Welfare Food Research Division, Bureau of Chemical Safety, found, for example, that cooked tomatoes contain ten to ninety times more ETU (fetus-deforming and cancer causing compound) than raw tomatoes from the same garden. His studies showed that ETU is the heat caused end product of widely used EBDC fungicides. He states, "Generally the amount of ETU in cooked vegetables was about 50 times more than in uncooked vegetables."

In animal experiments a classical study by Dr. F.M. Pottinger was conducted for ten years involving nine-hundred cats who were fed cooked and raw food diets. Results were observed for four generations. The cats fed cooked food developed the spectrum of degenerative diseases found in our society. In each succeeding generation, the disease became more chronic. By the third generation, reproduction became impossible. However, cats fed raw food continued to produce from one generation to the next healthy litters of youthful, flexible and active offsprings.

Most civilized people eat cooked food. Dr. Howell carried out extensive work to minimize the damage due to such dietary indulgence. He was the first researcher to investigate the digestive enzyme supplementation for the cooked food eating vegetarian as well as mixed diet user. He noted that pancreatin enzyme supplementation was useless in the high acid of the stomach since it functions best in the high alkaline environment of the small intestine. The papaine enzymes used in tenderizing meat needed high temperatures, beyond stomach range, so it was not fully potent as a supplement. Unripe papaya and pineapple work well on protein only. The best source of a mixture of digestive enzymes has been found in the different strains of the Aspergillus plants. They work on the full range of fats, proteins, carbohydrates and cellulose. Dr. Howell, in spite of doing the research and pioneer work on these most perfect enzymes, has maintained complete independence of any financial involvement with the manufacture and marketing of such products.

In my contacts in healing work, I have found that although many turned to raw foods for the alleviation of disease, the majority continued to maintain themselves on dead food, leading to eventual pain, stress and ailment. In an attempt to help them I saw that it was essential to have food thoroughly digested, the nutrients successfully distributed in cells, and fecal waste eliminated. This led to the supplement program of digestive enzymes, liquid chlorophyll and cayenne for circulation and a mild herbal for building up strength of internal organs so that effective elimination of waste and fecal matter could take place. As I searched for the perfect enzyme supplementation for those who still insist on using cooked food, and having experimented with most enzymes on the market, I found that the Aspergillus plant in capsules are best. Two to five capsules with the meal on food (preferably shaken out of the capsule) is best.

A good example of the potency of this approach was my Grandmother - a bedridden case of heart disease, asthma, arthritis, and kidney disorder of eighty years of age. Within several weeks of the inauguration of the supplementation program, she was doing all the house chores for a family of four, - cooking, laundry, cleaning, as well as reading, praying, watching television and socializing. From bed to full activity: this high energy continued for over two years.

A human is nourished and maintained not by what he eats, but by what is digested. All food is, at least potentially, a poison, until converted into simple structures by enzymes. There are two types of life building chemistries. One is found in raw food and called exogenous; the other is produced within your own body and is referred to as endogenous enzymes. The more enzymes one gets from exogenous sources like raw food, the less will have to be supplied by the pancreas and leukocytes, thus allowing endogenous enzymes to be utilized for the body maintenance, waste disposal, and extension of longevity. The enzymes found in raw food are released immediately after chewing to start breaking down the ingested food. Within thirty minutes after a meal, the acidity rises significantly and the ingested food enzymes become inactivated. Now the protein process takes over as it is acted upon by the hydrochloric acid and pepsin of the stomach.

There are more than 80,000 enzyme systems, each performing a specialized function from digestion of food to color of hair, to movement of the tongue or retina as you are speaking or reading this text. The food substances - protein, fats, carbohydrate, vitamin, mineral - are the raw materials which are utilized by the enzymes systems to carry on all the life processes and create all body parts.

You can eat a diet that has no enzymes and still live for many years, even to ripe old age, but through each generation you would produce inferior offspring, and eventually reproduction would be impossible. Would it not be better to let outside enzymes do some of the work and save your own enzymes for cellular work? It is possible that cellular enzyme exhaustion is the root cause of what ails us.

Dr. Howell and other researchers show that cooked food with the fiber broken down passes through the digestive system more slowly than raw foods. Partially, it ferments, rots, putrefies, throwing back into the body harmful substances, causing gas, heartburn and degenerative diseases.

Colon therapists and researchers in degenerative diseases have shown that much of the body weight can be just waste accumulated within the 60,000 miles of blood vessels, the lymphatic system, bone joint and intra-extra-cellular regions. The largest amount is found in the impactations within the colon structures: fecal waste can add up to an accumulated fifty pounds over the decades from feasting on greasy food. Due to the presence of this partially digested cooked food along the small intestine and colon, some of it passes into the bloodstream and is deposited as waste throughout the system. If it is calories, it can show up as obesity; if excess minerals we have arthritis; excess protein is built into cancer; fat leads to high cholesterol; sugar to diabetes.

The best alternatives to cooked and chemicalized foods is growing organic produce seasonally, purchasing additional food from natural method growers and starting a home indoor program of the high enzyme foods; soaked seeds, sprouts, baby greens, milk or ferment products from soaked seeds or nuts, raw foods, rejuvilac and raw juices.

Most people do not seem to have a large variance of vitamins and minerals over the years. However, the enzyme levels drop significantly in aging; as the body gets weaker and the enzymes get fewer, old age symptoms manifest. At the world famous Michael Reese Hospital in Chicago, researchers found that old people have only one- thirtieth as much enzymes in the saline as young folks. Also people with high enzymes diets have extensive longevity patterns. For example, people like Georgians, Ecuadorians, and Hunzas have diets rich in enzymes and have a high concentration of centurions (*National Geographic*, June 1973). They make extensive use of fermentation - soy, dairy, vegetables and fruits. Also, they utilize sprouting as well as soaking of seeds which increases the enzyme level up to twenty times and raw or undercooked food. They also fast seasonally during periods of food scarcity. Dr. Howell states that during fasting there is a halt in digestive enzyme production. The enzymes are used to digest the partially digested stored food of fatty tissue, scars, arthritis, tumor, hardening of the arteries, etc. Thus, the enforced fast is another health and longevity promoting benefit.

Dr. Howell's contribution to our understanding of enzymes and raw food research shows that not only will the physical man be healed, but also the spiritual being will manifest. He provides the evidence that cooked food contributes to the pathological over-enlargement of the pituitary gland, which regulates the other glands. In a study of accidental deaths where the victims aged over fifty, it was found that one hundred percent of them had a defective pituitary. The gonads, adrenals, isles of Langerhans and other ductless glands of most folks are exhausted from cooked food. These are the spiritual energy organs.

Raw food can assist you to be intuitive, high in *prana*, and in communion with God.

Dr. Howell's classic work on enzymes precedes the discovery of biological transmutation by Louis Kervan who showed that enzymes are actively involved in the alchemy of converting one element into another. A diet which centers on cooked foods leads to enzymes exhaustion and the impossibility of transmutation. The existence of people in the past, as well as now who eat or drink *nothing*, but who nevertheless carry on normal high energy lives, shows that the human system, when not having to eliminate waste can become a complete ecosystem with recycling and transmutation monitored such that the only input required is air and sunlight and a lifestyle free of all emotional stress, that is, a life of love and service.

The superiority of the raw food diet over cooked food can be tested in many new ways. Kinesiology, which utilizes strength change in the muscle and organ systems is one method. Have the individual stand with right arm (opposite for left handed) extended straight out, parallel to the ground, palm up. Test arm strength by pulling down on wrist. Next test the following procedure. Place in your left palm against the solar plexus separately a processed carbohydrate (sugar), cooked carbohydrate (bread), soaked wheat, sprouted sunflower, baby sunflower greens, sunflower yogurt, and finally sunflower cheese. You will be amazed at the strength generated by raw food, especially sprouted or fermented food, in comparison to the cooked versions. As this food stays in your body twelve to twenty-four hours, it will be likewise strengthening or weakening your body.

Chromatography is another method. This technique has been used in urine analysis up to 1944. In 1953, Dr. E. Pfeiffer used it to test for qualitative and biological values that give indications of enzyme activity. The chromatograph is a picture of color, rings and spike-like forms with a definite pattern that shows enzyme presence. Inorganic minerals, chemicals, or synthetic vitamins and cooked produce showed only colored rings but no definite pattern.

Most folks can demonstrate the enzyme action of ptyalin in the mouth by chewing an unsweetened slice of whole wheat bread. In no time it turns sweet in the mouth. Also, in high school, students use a simple test to demonstrate the presence of starch. By adding one drop of tincture of iodine to starch mixture, a blue color will result. If one teaspoon of starch mixture clears, then the iodine will cause no color change. The starch has been converted to maltose, a form of sugar.

Now on the market is available a thermography machine (AGA Company, 550 County Avenue, Secaucus, New Jersey 07094) which creates photos based on the heat generated by body cells, which depend on the free flow of nutrients and oxygen. The comparative photos that I have done show a clear facial image in the photo of a raw foodist, high enzyme eater. However, the photos of old people or young people on cooked food diet create images that are totally devoid of detail, thus indicating poor circulation and a badly starved body.

With this advancement in technology and the development of new methods of testing, the work of Dr. Howell stands uncontradicted. "*The Status of Food Enzymes in Digestion and Metabolism*" may be the most important book in scientific nutrition that has been written by a doctor and published in this century. Its range is beyond everyone else's and it makes the subject an exciting challenge. Dr. Howell shows that you can create your own health environment through dietary choice, raw foods in preference to cooked. Given the time, we will see that the man was a genius, creating forty years ago a nutritional theory that will be instrumental in healing degenerative disorders, extending longevity, and delineating some of the physiology of higher states of consciousness. I feel that 1981 will be the "Year of the Enzyme" and the 1980's will be the decade when raw foods will be considered the most important component in one's diet.

Victoras Kulvinskas, M.S.

Woodstock Valley, Connecticut
November 6, 1980

AN EXCLUSIVE INTERVIEW
with pioneer food enzyme researcher
DR. EDWARD HOWELL

Dr. Edward Howell was born in Chicago in 1898. He is the holder of a limited medical license from the State of Illinois.

The holder of a limited practice license is required to pass the same medical examination as a medical doctor. Only surgery, obstetrics and materia medica are excluded.

After obtaining his license, Dr. Howell joined the professional staff of the Lindlahr Sanitarium, where he remained for six years. In 1930, he established a private facility for the treatment of chronic ailments by nutritional and physical methods.

Until he retired in 1970, Dr. Howell was busy in private practice three days each week. The balance of his time he devoted to various kinds of research.

Dr. Howell is the first researcher to recognize the importance of the enzymes in food to human nutrition. In 1946, he wrote the book, *The Status of Food Enzymes in Digestion and Metabolism.*

This book contains the reference and source materials for the enzyme theories which Dr. Howell has collectively called, *"The Food Enzyme Concept."* The manuscript was republished in 1980 under the title *Food Enzymes for Health & Longevity.* In 1985 *Enzyme Nutrition* by Dr. Howell was published. This manuscript reviews the scientific literature and presents food enzymes as essential nutrients.

In this interview, Dr. Howell tells: What enzymes are, what they do in our bodies, why he believes a state of enzyme deficiency stress exists in most people, and finally, what he believes you can do about it.

What are enzymes?

Enzymes are substances which make life possible. They are needed for every chemical reaction that occurs in our body. Without enzymes, no activity at all would take place. Neither vitamins, minerals or hormones can do any work without enzymes.

Think of it this way: Enzymes are the *"labor force"* that builds your body just like construction workers are the labor force that builds your house. You may have all the necessary building materials and lumber, but to build a house you need workers, which represent the vital life elements.

Similarly, you may have all the nutrients - vitamins, proteins, minerals, etc., for your body, but you still need the *enzymes - the life element* - to keep the body alive and well.

Are enzymes then just like chemical catalysts which speed up various reactions?

No. Enzymes are much more than catalysts.

Catalysts are only inert substances. They possess none of the life energy we find in enzymes. For instance, enzymes give off a kind of radiation when they work. This is not true of catalysts. In addition, although enzymes contain proteins - and some contain vitamins - the activity factor of enzymes has never been synthesized.

Moreover, there is no combination of proteins or any combination of amino acids or any other substance which will give enzyme activity. There are proteins present in enzymes. However, they serve only as carriers of the enzyme activity factors.

Therefore, we can say that enzymes consist of protein carriers charged with energy factors just as a battery consists of metallic plates charged with electrical energy.

Where do the enzymes in our bodies come from?

It seems that we inherit a certain enzyme potential at birth.

This limited supply of activity factors of life force must last us a lifetime. It's just as if you inherited a certain amount of money. If the movement is all one way - all spending and no income you will run out of money.

Likewise, the faster you use up your supply of enzyme activity, the quicker you will run out. Experiments at various universities have shown that, regardless of the species, the faster the metabolic rate, the shorter the life-span.

Other things being equal, *you live as long as your body has enzyme activity factors to make enzymes from.* When it gets to the point that you can't make certain enzymes, then your life ends.

Do people do anything which causes them to waste their limited enzyme supply?

Yes. Just about every single person eats a diet of mainly cooked foods. Keep in mind that whenever a food is heated *at 212 degrees,* the *enzymes* in it are 100% *destroyed.*

If enzymes were in the food we eat, they would do some or even a considerable part of the work of digestion by themselves. However, when you eat cooked, enzyme-free food, this forces the body itself to make the enzymes needed for digestion. This depletes the body's limited enzyme capacity.

How serious is this strain on our enzyme "bank" caused by diets of mostly cooked food?

I believe it's *one of the paramount causes of premature aging and early death.* I also believe it's the underlying cause of almost all *degenerative disease.*

To begin with, if the body is overburdened to supply many enzymes to the saliva, gastric juice, pancreatic juice and intestinal juice, then it must curtail the production of enzymes for other purposes. If this occurs, then how can the body also make enough enzymes to run the brain, heart, kidneys, lungs, muscles and other organs and tissues?

This "stealing" of enzymes from other parts of the body to service the digestive tract sets up a competition for enzymes among the various organ systems and tissues of the body.

The resulting *metabolic dislocations may be the direct cause of cancer, coronary heart disease, diabetes, and many other chronic incurable diseases.*

This state of enzyme deficiency stress exists in the majority of persons on the civilized, enzyme-free diet.

Did human disease begin when man started cooking his food?

This is what the evidence indicates.

For example, the Neanderthal Man of 50,000 years ago used fire extensively in his cooking. He lived in caves and ate mostly roasted meat from the continuous fires which warmed the caves. These statements are documented by scientific evidence in my published and unpublished works.

From fossil evidence, we know that the Neanderthal Man suffered from fully-developed crippling arthritis.

It's possible that the Neanderthal Man also had diabetes or cancer or kidney disease and so forth. However, we'll never know since all soft tissues have disappeared without a trace.

Incidentally, another inhabitant of the caves was the cave bear. This creature protected the Neanderthal Man from the cave tiger, who also wanted the protection of the cave to avoid the frigid weather. The cave bear, according to paleontologists, was a partially domesticated animal and most likely lived on the same roasted meat that the cave man ate.

Like the cave man, the cave bear also suffered from chronic, deforming arthritis.

Isn't it possible that cold weather, not cooked food, was responsible for the arthritis of the Neanderthal Man?

No, I don't think weather had much to do with it. For example, consider the primitive Eskimo. He lived in an environment just as frigid as that of the Neanderthal Man. And yet, the *Eskimo never suffered from arthritis and other chronic diseases.* However, the Eskimo ate large amounts of *raw food.* The meat he ate was only slightly heated and was raw in the center. Therefore, the Eskimo received a large quantity of food enzymes with every meal. In fact, the word Eskimo itself comes from an Indian expression which means, "He who eats it raw."

Incidentally, there is no tradition of medicine men among the Eskimo people. But among groups like the North American Indian, who ate cooked food extensively, the medicine man had a prominent position in the tribe.

What evidence is there that human beings suffer from food enzyme deficiency?

There's so much evidence that I can only briefly summarize a small fraction of it. Over the last 40 years, I have collected thousands of scientific documents to substantiate my theories.

To begin with, human beings have the lowest levels of starch digesting enzymes in their blood of any creature. We also have the highest level of these enzymes in the urine, meaning that they are being used up faster.

There's other evidence showing that these low enzyme levels are not due to a peculiarity of our species. Instead, they are due to the large amounts of cooked starch we eat.

Also, we know that decreased enzyme levels are found in a number of chronic ailments, such as allergies, skin disease, and even serious diseases like diabetes and cancer.

In addition, incriminating evidence indicates that cooked, enzyme-free diets contribute to a pathological over-enlargement of the pituitary gland, which regulates the other glands. Furthermore, there is documented research showing that almost 100% of the people over 50, dying from accidental causes were found to have defective pituitary glands.

Next, I believe that *food enzyme deficiency is the cause of the exaggerated maturation of today's children and teenagers.* It is also an important cause of overweight in many children and adults.

Many animal experiments have shown that enzyme-deficient diets produce a much more rapid maturation than usual. Animals on cooked diets are also much heavier than their counter-parts on raw diets. Another piece of related evidence is that farmers use cooked potatoes to fatten pigs for market. They've found that pigs on cooked potatoes fatten faster and more economically than pigs on raw potatoes.

This evidence shows the great difference between cooked calories and raw calories. Indeed, from my work in a sanitarium many years ago, I've found that *it was impossible to get people fat on raw foods, regardless of the calorie intake.*

Incidentally, another effect associated with *food enzyme deficiency* is that the *size of the brain decreases.* In addition, the thyroid over-enlarges, even in the presence of adequate iodine. This has been shown in a number of species. Of course, you can't prove it on human beings. The evidence, however, is very suggestive.

What else is there?

Next, consider that the *human pancreas is burdened with enzyme production far in excess* of any creature living on a raw food diet. In fact, in proportion to body weight, the human pancreas is more than twice as heavy as that of a cow.

Human beings eat mainly cooked food, while cows eat raw grass.

Then, there is evidence that rats on a cooked diet have a pancreas about twice as heavy as rats on a raw diet.

Moreover, evidence shows that the human pancreas is one of the heaviest in the animal kingdom, when you adjust for total body weight.

This *over-enlargement of the human pancreas is just as dangerous - probably even more so - than an over-enlargement of the heart, the thyroid and so on.* The overproduction of enzymes in humans is a pathological adaptation to a diet of enzyme-free foods.

The pancreas is not the only part of the body that over-secretes enzymes when the diet is cooked. In addition, there are the human salivary glands, which produce enzymes to a degree never found in wild animals on their natural foods.

In fact, some animals on a raw diet do not have any enzymes at all in their saliva. The cow and sheep produce torrents of saliva with no enzymes in it.

Dogs, for instance, also secrete no enzymes in their saliva when they're eating a raw diet. However, if you start giving them cooked starchy food, their salivary glands will start producing starch-digesting enzymes within 10 days.

In addition, there's more evidence that the enzymes in saliva represent a pathological and not a normal situation. To begin with, salivary enzymes cannot digest raw starch. This is something I demonstrated in the laboratory.

The enzymes in saliva will only attack a piece of starch once it's cooked. Therefore, we see that the body will channel some of its limited enzyme producing capacity into saliva only if it has to. Incidentally, there is some provocative animal research which I have done in my own laboratory some years ago. If you'd like, I can explain it now for you readers.

Yes, please do.

I fed one group of rats a cooked diet and one group a raw diet and let them live out their life-span to see which group would live longer.

The first group got a combination of raw meat and various raw vegetables and grains. The second group got the same foods boiled and therefore enzyme-free. I kept these rats until they died, which took about three years.

As the experiment came to a close, the results surprised me. It turned out that there was no great difference between the life-spans of the two groups. Later on, I discovered the reason.

It turned out that the rats on the cooked diet were still getting enzymes, but from an unexpected source. They had been eating their own feces, which contained the enzymes excreted from their own bodies.

All feces, including those of human beings, contain the enzymes that the body has used. My rats had been recycling their own enzymes to use them over again. And that's why they lived as long as the rats on the raw diet.

Incidentally, the practice of eating feces is almost universal among today's laboratory animals. Although these animals receive "scientific" diets containing all known vitamins and minerals, the animals instinctively know they need enzymes. Because of this, they eat their own feces.

In fact, the *animals on these scientific diets develop most of the chronic human degenerative diseases if they are allowed to live out their life-spans. This shows that vitamins and minerals alone are not sufficient for health.*

How do you know that people would benefit from additional enzyme intake?

To me, the most impressive evidence that people need enzymes is what occurs as a result of therapeutic fasting. As you know, I spent some years in a sanitarium working with patients on various fasting programs.

When a person fasts, there is an immediate halt to the production of digestive enzymes. The enzymes in saliva, gastric juice and pancreatic juice dwindle and become scarce. *During fasting, the body's enzymes are free to work on repairing and removing diseased tissues.*

Civilized people eat such large quantities of cooked foods that their enzyme systems are kept busy digesting food. As a result, the body lacks the enzymes needed to maintain the tissues in good health. Most people who fast go through what is called a healing crisis. The patients may feel nausea, vomiting and dizziness. What's happening is that the enzymes are working to change the unhealthy structure of the body. The enzymes attack pathological tissues and break down undigested and unprocessed substances; and these then get thrown out through the bowels, through vomiting, or via the skin.

When people get enzymes from food, aren't they destroyed by stomach acid and therefore of little or no value?

This is not true. Although most nutritionists claim that enzymes in food are destroyed in the stomach, they overlook two important facts.

First of all, when you eat food, acid secretion is minimal for at least thirty minutes. As the food goes down the esophagus, it drops into the top portion of the stomach. This is called the cardiac section, since it's closer to the heart.

The rest of the stomach remains flat and closed while the cardiac section opens up to accommodate the food. *During the time the food sits in the upper section,* little acid or enzymes are secreted by the body. *The enzymes in the food itself go about digesting the food.* The more of this self-digestion , the less work the body has to do later.

When this 30 to 45 minute period is over, the bottom section of the stomach opens up and the body starts secreting acid and enzymes. Even at this point, the food enzymes are not inactivated until the acid level becomes prohibitive. You see, food enzymes can tolerate chemical environments many times more acid than neutral.

Do animals also have a special section of the stomach where food digests itself?

Absolutely. In fact, some creatures have what I call a food enzyme stomach.

There are the cheek pouches of monkeys and rodents, the crop of many species of birds, and the first stomachs of whales, dolphins and porpoises.

When birds, for instance, swallow seeds or grains, these grains lie in the crop for 8 to 12 hours. As they sit, they absorb moisture, swell up and begin to germinate. During germination, enzymes are formed which do the work of digesting the seeds and grains.

Whales, dolphins and porpoises have a first stomach which secretes no enzymes. Whales, for example, swallow large quantities of food without chewing it. The food simply decomposes and digests itself. In the flesh of the fish and other marine life the whale eats is an enzyme called cathepsin, which breaks down the fish once it has died. In fact, this enzyme is present in almost all creatures.

After the whale's catch has liquefied itself, it passes through a small hole into the whale's second stomach.

It mystifies scientists how the whale's catch can get through that small hole into the second stomach. They have no idea that self-digestion is at work.

Most - if not all of us, eat lots of cooked foods every day. Can we make up for this enzyme loss by eating raw foods in addition?

No. Cooked foods are such a large drain on our enzyme supply that you can't make it up by eating raw foods.

In addition, vegetables and fruits are not concentrated sources of enzymes. When produce ripens, enzymes are present to do the ripening. However, once the ripening is finished, some of the enzymes leave and go back into the stem and seeds.

For example, when companies want to get enzymes from papaya, a tropical fruit, they use the juice of unripe papaya. The ripe papaya itself has no great concentration of enzymes.

Are there any foods particularly high in enzymes?

Bananas, avocados and mangoes are good sources. In general, foods having a higher calorie content are richer in enzymes.

Do you recommend all raw foods as sources of enzymes?

No. There are some foods, seeds and nuts, that contain what are called enzyme inhibitors.

These enzyme inhibitors are present for the protection of the seed. Nature doesn't want the seed to germinate prematurely and lose its life. It wants to make sure that the seed is present in soil with sufficient moisture to grow and continue the species.

Therefore, when you eat raw seeds or raw nuts, you are swallowing enzyme inhibitors which will neutralize some of the enzymes your body produces. In fact, eating foods with enzyme inhibitors causes a swelling of the pancreas.

All nuts and seeds contain these inhibitors. Raw peanuts, for example, contain an especially large amount. Raw wheat germ is also one of the worst offenders. In addition, all peas, beans and lentils contain some.

Potatoes, which are seeds, have enzyme inhibitors.

In eggs, which are also seeds, the inhibitor is contained mainly in the egg-white.

As a general rule, enzyme inhibitors are confined to the seed portions of food. For instance, the eyes of potatoes. The inhibitors are not present in the fleshy portions of fruits or in the leaves and stems of vegetables.

There are two ways to destroy enzyme inhibitors. The first is cooking, however, this also destroys the enzymes. The second way, which is preferable, is *sprouting*. This *destroys the enzyme inhibitors and also increases the enzyme content by a factor of 3 to 6.*

Some foods, like soybeans, must be especially well heated to destroy the inhibitors. For example, many of the soy flours and powders on the market are not heated enough to destroy the inhibitors.

There is one other way to neutralize enzyme inhibitors, but we'll get to it in just a minute.

You said that it's not possible to overcome the enzyme drain of cooked foods just by eating other raw foods. What then can people do?

The only solution is to take *capsules of concentrated plant enzymes.*

In the absence of contraindications, you should take from 1 to 3 capsules per meal. Of course, if you are eating all raw foods, then no enzymes will be necessary at that meal.

The capsules should be opened and sprinkled on the food or chewed with the meal. This way, the enzymes can go to work immediately. Incidentally, taking extra enzymes is the third way to neutralize the enzyme inhibitors in unsprouted seeds and nuts.

Concentrates of plant enzymes or fungus enzymes are better for predigestion of food than tablets of pancreatic enzymes. This is because plant enzymes can work in the acidity of the stomach, whereas pancreatic enzymes only work best in the alkalinity of the small intestine.

If the enzyme tablet has an enteric coating, then it's not suitable, since it will only release after it has passed the stomach. By this time, it's too late for food predigestion. The body itself has already used its own enzymes to digest the food.

Would people benefit from taking enzymes, even if they have no problem with diges-tion or if they eat mainly raw foods?

They probably would benefit. Our bodies use up enzymes in so many ways that *it pays to maintain your enzyme bank,* regardless of what you eat.

For example, enzymes are used up faster during certain illnesses, during extremely hot or cold weather, and during strenuous exercise.

Also, keep in mind that any enzymes that are taken are not wasted since they add to the enzyme pool of your body.

Furthermore, as we pass our prime, the amount of enzymes in our bodies and excreted in our sweat and urine continues to decline until we die. In fact, *low enzyme levels are associated with old age and chronic disease.*

So far, there's not much hard evidence on whether taking addi-tional enzymes will extend the life-span. However, we do know that *laboratory rats* that eat raw foods will live about 3 years. Rats that eat enzymeless chow diets will live only 2 years. Thus, we see that *diets deficient in enzymes cause a 30% reduction in life-span.*

If this held true for human beings, it may mean that people could extend their life-spans by 20 or more years - just by maintaining proper enzyme levels.

Chapter 1

ROLE OF FOOD ENZYMES IN NUTRITION

It is a dictum of science that man's early progenitors were similar to present day anthropoids in form and habit. The ancestors of man were not cooking animals. It is not difficult to imagine a time when early man must have consumed his food just as he found it, *untouched by fire*. When primitive man first became acquainted with the use of fire, cookery may have had its origin, but it was not the highly efficient art we know today. It is commonly taken for granted that because heat preparation of food has a long history, the practice must be above reproach as to any deleterious effect on human health. It might be argued that the human race could not have survived countless centuries of cookery if its effect on health was harmful. And yet, everyone is acquainted with the destructive nature of fire and high temperature.

But the complete adequacy of a diet is not to be judged solely by its ability to sustain reproduction. The *length of the life span and the incidence of degenerative diseases must also be considered*. If the human race were entirely free from degenerative diseases, the critical observer could choose to ignore the potentially destructive effects of cookery. But since this is not the case, and, furthermore, since the incidence of several degenerative and destructive diseases is increasing, it is a duty not to be shunned by anyone, to regard with utmost suspicion any and all significant departures from the living habits of the primitive ancestors of man.

The usual experiment calculated to determine the vitamin value of a diet occupies only a relatively short time in the total life span of the animal. The early growing period is utilized, whereas chronic degenerative diseases usually make their appearance at a later time in the life cycle. Pronouncements cannot be made that a synthetic diet with added salts and vitamins, which is effective in promoting normal increase in weight and normal reproduction in a young growing rat, will be equally effective in maintaining normal health in the latter half of the life span and in sponsoring a normal length of life. Those few experiments that have been conducted during the whole life time of rats, usually 2 to 4 years, have shown conclusively that rats cannot be maintained on the usual balanced synthetic diets without developing a variety of pathological conditions. McCay and associates (1) found that at least half of the rats living beyond 2 years became blind. Genito-urinary diseases were frequent. I take this up in greater detail later in the discussion.

I have a large volume of evidence relating that not only the temperatures used in cookery are highly destructive, but also that those even considerably below pasteurization kill many different enzymes. And it is a general opinion that such temperatures are destructive to all enzymes. In view of these facts, it can readily be seen that the average prepared meal bequeaths to its host only a negligible fraction of the enzymes present in the same food before being heat-treated. With these facts clearly in mind, it remains to be shown *whether food enzymes have a function to perform in the animal body.*

Enzymes, whether those present in food or in the digestive secretions, are highly active substances and commence to function as soon as conditions of temperature and moisture are suitable. When uncooked starchy food is eaten, a period of time transpires during which the food absorbs moisture. After the water content reaches a proper level, conditions immediately become congenial for the action of the food enzymes within the starch granules. Digestion has already started before the enzymes of the digestive fluids are poured out and begin the task. The stimulus for secretion of enzymes by the glands is only normally active and the quantity secreted is not excessive. The capacity for long continued secretion is thus conserved until old age. These points are considered in detail later.

In spite of the current tendency towards the use of more raw fruits and vegetables in the diet, I believe our agricultural forefathers got more enzymes in the old-fashioned diet. Present day rapid and highly efficient cookery is a procedure very different from the practice of former times. Some primitive peoples cook by placing heated stones into the food. Roasting is performed over an open fire. Such methods do not insure thorough penetration of the heat and it is questionable whether the enzymes not in immediate contact with the heat are destroyed. Stefansson (2) stated that the Eskimo does not practice frying and that when cooking is resorted to, it is an invariable rule to make it only of such duration that the interior of the meat remains rare. Bread was formerly often imperfectly baked, sometimes remaining partly raw inside. With modern automatic ovens, a temperature of 350 to 400 degrees F insures even and thorough penetration of the heat. Many foods are now fried and the temperature of frying is well over 300 degrees F. In past times, beer and wine were consumed unheated. Our agricultural forefathers used unheated honey, milk, cheese, and butter. Now all extracted honey is heated at 140 to 165 degrees F for 24 to 72 hours to prevent solidification. Whereas raw honey was formerly used more or less extensively, since the advent of inexpensive sugar, honey is not used to the same extent. Even fruit juices are being more and more taken from the can.

Granted that vegetables are good sources of many minerals and vitamins, they are, however, extremely low in enzyme content. For instance, as a result of tests I have made, it appears that the amylase activity of resting (ungerminated) wheat grains is more than 100 times greater than that of raw cabbage. Modern dietitians try to balance the diet by encouraging use of fresh, non-starchy vegetables, but this does not correct the diet for enzymes. Foods with high calorie values, such as bread and meat, although containing moderate amounts of enzymes to begin with, lose them during the culinary heat treatment. An attempt to balance such a diet by addition of fresh vegetables of low calorie value, adds only small amounts of enzymes, while large amounts have been removed during preparation. Since a vast proportion of the population satisfies the calorie requirements with heat-treated foods which retain little or none of the enzymes, it is seen that there is an astounding decrease in the enzyme intake.

The physical changes caused by heat in food cannot be considered as factors in making toward poor health and pathological developments. It might be argued that cooked food, being softer, is customarily gulped and insufficiently masticated, with a resulting strain upon the digestive mechanism. However, careful observers of the life of the primitive Eskimo, including Stefansson, agree that the Eskimo gulps his meat like a dog, without any mastication whatever. If insufficient mastication were to be considered accountable for major disturbances in health, then isolated Eskimos should logically display an incidence of dental caries, digestive disturbances, and other common diseases at least equivalent to our own. Such, I propose to show, is far from the case.

Chapter 2

INTESTINAL ABSORBABILITY OF ENZYMES

Because enzymes do not pass through the intestinal membrane *in vitro* (laboratory culture), the assumption has become general that enzymes cannot be absorbed from the intestinal canal during life. In experiments on the passage of various sugars through the intestinal wall *in vivo* (in living organism) and *in vitro*, the physiologist Westenbrink (3) achieved opposite results and concluded that gut permeability *in vitro* has little resemblance to absorption *in vivo*. That various substances, including undigested proteins, can be absorbed into the circulation is now established. Shuger and Arnold (4), Research Laboratories, Illinois Dept. of Public Health, University of Illinois, have shown that culture of *B. prodigiosus, B. murii* and *B. welchii* was successful and the organisms recoverable from the mesenteric lymph gland, liver, spleen, and lungs of dogs, if the animals were killed within 15 minutes after placing the bacteria into the lumen of the large intestine. The organs of dogs killed one hour after rectal injection of bacteria were all free of viable bacteria. The 30 and 45 minutes intervals after rectal injection showed progressively fewer bacteria in the organs cultured as compared to the 15 minute time interval. Sixteen dogs were used as controls. Rats also were used and the observations on dogs substantiated. This work suggests that in experiments designed to determine whether enzymes are absorbable, the time at which a blood sample is taken may be the determining factor between positive and negative results.

Fisher (5), Dept. of Bacteriology, University of Illinois, determined that one cake of Fleischmann's compressed yeast fed to dogs by stomach tube, produced positive yeast cultures in the liver, lymph glands, lungs, spleen, and kidneys, proving that the whole yeast cells were absorbed into the circulation from the lumen of the intestine. In later experiments, Fisher (6) showed that injection of yeast cells into the colon of dogs is followed, as with bacteria, by absorption and recovery of the live yeast by culture, in the organs, the greatest recovery being at the 15 minute period and diminishing thereafter until none could be demonstrated at the two-hour interval. The fact that bacteria and yeast cells were found in lymph tissues is important in emphasizing the mechanism of absorption. Tychowski (7) traced the absorption of Chinese ink from a loop of intestine in the rabbit and the dog, and observed particles of it in the lymphatics, in the bodies of the leukocytes, and in small veins. He witnessed that the leukocytes are the carriers of the ink.

Alexander and associates (8), Dept. of Internal Medicine, Washington University School of Medicine, were readily able to show by precipitation tests, the presence of egg white in lymph from the thoracic duct, but not in the portal blood. They concluded that the route of ingested protein to the systemic circulation is via the thoracic duct lymph. Egg white was fed to dogs by stomach tube. Several independent investigations have established the fact that unchanged proteins may be absorbed from the intestine. Ratner (9), New York University, stated that the passage of native protein through the intact wall is physiological and occurs with greater regularity than is generally believed. Ratner and Gruehl (10) offer as conclusive evidence that unsplit protein can be absorbed unchanged through the walls of the intestine, the fact that mature and young animals can be sensitized and shocked by oral administration of proteins. Wilson and Walzer (11) believe the absorption of unaltered egg protein to be normal physiological function in infants and children, as well as adults. The former view that enzymes cannot be absorbed because they are colloidal, cannot, therefore, be sustained, since many complex substances such as bacteria, yeast cells, and proteins can pass through the walls of the intestine.

The most painstaking effort yet put forth in attempting to find out whether enzymes can be absorbed from the intestine, is the work of Crandall (12), Northwestern University. A number of dogs were prepared with jejunal and Eck fistulae and after recovery received fresh active pancreatic juice or human saliva by way of the jejunal fistula. Tests were made upon the blood serum for amylase and lipase, 1 hour, 2 hours, 4 hours, and 6 hours after administration of the enzymes. One of the faults of this technique is that there is no evidence that the blood serum is the proper medium to look for absorbed enzymes; in fact the overwhelming weight of evidence is to the contrary. Crandall could detect only a small increase in the serum enzyme level in some of the experiments after administration of the enzymes, and concluded that it is probable that small amounts of enzymes can be absorbed.

On the other hand, Oelgoetz and associates (13) have determined that when patients with low level of serum amylase are given 50 grains of extract of whole pancreas, the serum amylase level will be restored to normal within one hour and remain normal for approximately three days after which it gradually falls to the original level. If given to a normal individual, the serum amylase level remains unchanged; likewise, the concentration of amylase in the feces is unchanged. In order to determine what becomes of the ingested enzymes, Oelgoetz daily fed 30 grains of pancreatic extract each to a group of rabbits for one week. The animals were then sacrificed and extracts of the liver and spleen compared with controls for degree of amylase activity. It was found that *those rabbits receiving pancreatic extract had approximately twice as much liver amylase and 17 times as much amylase in the spleen as the rabbits used for controls.* Oelgoetz believes that the presence of a proper level of serum enzymes is an effective protection against food allergy occasioned by absorption of whole proteins and that a low serum enzyme level induces allergy. According to the experience of Oelgoetz and associates (14,15,16), when doses of pancreatic enzymes larger than the official doses are administered to patients having symptoms of allergy including a low serum enzyme level, the serum enzyme level returns to normal and the symptoms of allergy subside.

Virtanen and Soumalainen (17) gave subcutaneous injections of large amounts of pig pancreas lipase to guinea pigs and found most of the enzyme was retained, the greatest storage occurring in the liver. The same result followed in rabbits.

The serum enzymes, according to Oelgoetz and associates, provide the means whereby unsplit proteins, carbohydrates, and fats, gaining entrance to the blood stream, are broken down into simpler units and allergy thereby avoided. It is Oelgoetz's thesis that the blood stream provides an ideal environment as to constant pH, salt concentration, and temperature, for the completion, as a normal physiological process, of the digestion of adventitious and partly digested materials. A low serum enzyme level does not provide this protection. These authors have shown that functional digestive disturbances, gastric neuroses, hyperacidity, urticaria, and many gastrointestinal symptoms are readily relieved in individuals displaying a low serum enzyme index, when 15 grains of an extract of whole pancreas is administered three times daily. *Massive doses of enzymes*, in excess of the official recommendations, have been shown also, by other trustworthy clinicians, to be *effective in relieving certain digestive symptoms and a variety of dermatoses* thought to be due to irritation of the skin caused by the presence of incompletely digested food materials.

Boldyreff (18), by preparing dogs with fistulae at the beginning, middle, and end of the small intestine, claims to have observed, during the fasting state, that periodically secreted pancreatic and intestinal juices, including their enzymes, are entirely absorbed from the intestine into the blood, increasing the proteolytic and lipolytic properties of the blood.

Sansum (19), Potter Metabolic Clinic, Santa Barbara, California, regularly obtained a high percentage of favorable responses in indigestion, abdominal gas, food eczema, urticaria, and other conditions with massive doses of enzymes. The degree of response may be judged from the following table:

Number of Cases		*Number Improved*
34	Bronchial Asthma	88%
12	Food Asthma	92%
42	Food Eczema	83%
19	Hay Fever	80%
11	Loose Bowels	100%
54	Normal Weight	Remained constant
29	Overweight	93%
197	Underweight	91%
29	Urticaria or hives	86%

Sansum found fungus amylase to be efficient for relieving abdominal gas and employed it along with pepsin and pancreatin. Renda (20) reported improvement in 75 cases of certain forms of eczema in infants after use of large doses (8 to 50 grains) of dried whole pancreas in tablet or powder form for a period of one to four weeks.

Elson (21) believes psoriasis belongs to a class of enzyme-deficiency diseases, and that the patch consists of and is brought about by an outpouring and exuding - actually a purging as he calls it - of protein substances and some lipoids in various stages of digestion. During a period of 19 years, Elson has had remarkable success with psoriasis by administering massive doses of pancreatin (90 to 120 grains daily). The treatment occupies several months and Elson employed it in addition to other appropriate temporary treatment with marked success also in many ill-defined cases of eczema, many dermatoses of unknown origin, and many cases of food allergy.

I have been fortunate in finding a paper by Sellei (22,23), Chief of the Dermatological Section of the Hungarian State Railway Hospital, Budapest, Hungary, who discovered that enzyme therapy in skin afflictions is followed by slow improvement and even after being discontinued, this improvement continues. The Hungarian dermatologist recommended large quantities of enzymes - 8 to 10 pancreatin tablets and 100 to 150 grams raw pancreas daily. *Scleroderma verum* responded favorably to enzyme therapy; 90% of the cases investigated by the Rona-Michaelis test (atoxyl lipase resistance test) showed what Sellei described as pancreatic insufficiency. He reports 17 cases of various other skin afflictions in which good results were obtained as well as in other forms of what he calls dysfermatosis. Sellei claims that the remedies do not act in scleroderma merely by substitution, since, even when they are discontinued for a long period, there is no recurrence of the scleroderma. He continues: "After a few weeks of continuous treatment, a positive atoxyl lipase resistance in scleroderma verum becomes negative, which helps to prove the importance of these enzymes in relation to the entire organism. If enzyme therapy is given up, the atoxyl lipase resistance becomes positive again in these patients."

This provides strong evidence in favor of Oelgoetz's finding that a surplus of ingested enzymes is stored as a *reserve*, principally in the spleen and liver, to be drawn upon when required. The fact that certain afflictions of the skin can be regularly subdued through oral administration of enzymes, coupled with the fact that simultaneously with this improvement the serum enzyme level is raised from a low to a normal value, *proves* that enzymes can be absorbed from the intestinal tract in considerable and useful amounts.

What I believe is one of the most outstanding researches so far recorded on the fate of enzymes when taken orally was undertaken by Masumizu (24), Medical Clinic, Tohoku Imperial University, Japan. Masumizu's work is remarkable in several ways. The experiments were conducted, not upon isolated specimens of urine, but upon the complete 24 hour excretion, thereby insuring the presence of all enzymes excreted, instead of only a portion. The experimental animals, 10 rabbits, were given by *os*, 5 grams of pancreatin or 5 grams of fungus amylase for each rabbit per day. Since this dosage is comparatively enormous for small animals, the experiments prove beyond doubt that even large quantities of enzymes can be absorbed and find their way into the urine. Although Masumizu proved that the urinary excretion of amylase was approximately doubled when the enzymes were given, he was unable to secure any increase in the serum amylase concentration at all. He remarks that in all his experiments the level of amylase in the serum always remained constant and his figures bear out this contention. This confirms the observation of Oelgoetz who likewise found the serum amylase level uninfluenced by ingested enzymes unless it was below physiological limits.

I believe it is a tactical error to try testing the possibility of enzyme absorption through the intestine by examination of blood serum. Evidently these enzymes are not carried to the kidneys through blood serum. I will show the mechanism of their transport in subsequent discussion. I propose to prove that the normal channel for absorption of enzymes, as well as with proteins, is through the lymph. Masumizu's technique involved collection of 24 hour urine specimens for a period of 5 to 10 days. The total daily amylase excretion was calculated by daily test of the urine, and the sum total of the daily values established the amylase excretion value which served as a control figure. The same animal was then given pancreatin or fungus amylase, the urine collected, and the amylase value determined for a similar period. The fungus enzyme had an amylase value about 10 times higher than that of the pancreatin used, which was a product of Parke Davis & Co. In all experiments with fungus amylase, the amylolytic power of the urine was more than doubled. The amount of the enzyme excreted comprised a large proportion of what was administered. But in the case of pancreatin, the proportion of excreted enzyme was even greater, compared to the amount taken in, than when fungus amylase was used.

It might seem possible that enzymes are less liable to suffer destruction in passing through the stomach of the rabbit than would be the case with carnivorous or mixed feeders. This, however, is not the case. According to various investigators the average pH of the stomach contents of several species is as follows:

Rabbit	1 to 2
Man	1 to 2
Rat	3 to 4
Dog	3 to 4

According to these figures the stomach of the dog, as an example, offers a more congenial environment for pancreatic enzymes than that of the rabbit. Thus Masumizu's experiments cannot be invalidated on the supposition that the stomach of the herbivorous rabbit is not destructive to enzymes, since it is evident that the acid concentration of the rabbit's stomach is high.

Enzyme intake of such magnitude that the organism cannot promptly use or store is eliminated by a mechanism similar to that of regulating excretion of water intake in excess of the storage capacity or needs of the tissues. If the blood stream is overloaded with absorbed enzymes, the storage capacity of the tissues is momentarily overtaxed and the enzymes are eliminated through the urine, in much the same way as a sudden excess of sugar or water is eliminated in the urine.

But because there may still remain doubt as to whether the absorption of enzymes in large quantities is a normal, physiologic occurrence, I shall proceed with further recitation of important facts. Kallo (25,26), Pathology Institute, Royal Hungarian Franz-Joseph University, Szeged, compared the lipolytic activity of the lymph of the *cisterna chyli* with that of the blood of the *vena cava* inferior and of the *vena portae* in 21 dogs. The lymph usually contained a much larger amount of lipase than the blood, especially when a fat-rich diet was used. Kallo concluded that these lipases may be absorbed from the abdominal organs, pancreas, liver, and intestinal tract in two ways: (a) directly through the lymph vessels of these organs, or (b) indirectly following previous introduction into the intestinal tract by the pancreatic or intestinal juice.

Kokuryo (27) claimed maltase of the blood and urine originates partly from the pancreas and partly from the intestine.

Chapter 3

COMPARATIVE NORMAL ENZYME VALUE OF BODY FLUIDS

Cohen (28) found that the output of amylase in the urine varied greatly, with an immediate rise after a meal, and thought that amylase is irregularly absorbed from the gut. The blood amylase remained at a constant level despite marked changes in urinary amylase content, thus confirming the findings of Oelgoetz and Masumizu. Cameron (29) showed that the urinary amylase follows a regular cycle of rise and fall intimately connected with the digestive process. After a meal, the amylolytic power reaches a relatively high value - in some cases within a very short interval, such as half an hour; in others more gradually, the maximum usually being reached within one to two hours after the meal.

In an extensive study of urinary amylase excretion, Eckhardt (30), State Hospital, Plauen, Germany, showed that it varied with food consumption. Reid (31) examined specimens of urine every hour for amylase content and found it highest in the period of the second to the fifth hour after meals; thereafter the value tends to fall.

On the other hand, it has been repeatedly demonstrated, by Carlson and Luckhardt, University of Chicago (32); Wohlgemuth, Pathology Institute, University of Berlin (33); Kleinmann and Scharr (34), and others, that the blood serum enzymes remain constant in health and bear no relation to food or meals. Kleinmann and Scharr determined the proteases cathepsin and trypsin in the blood serum of rabbits. The values were remarkably constant, varying not more than 5 to 7 per cent. Furthermore, the serum enzyme content seemed to be independent of whether the blood was taken from fasting rabbits or immediately after feeding. Wohlgemuth found that variations in the diet, both in the kind of food and in the amount, have no immediate effect upon the amylase content of the blood serum.

Professor Carlson once stated: "If the blood diastase is pancreatic amylopsin resorbed from the alimentary tract, it would seem natural to find more of the ferment in the blood of herbivora than in the blood of carnivora, and again, we might reasonably look for an increase in a carnivorous animal when kept on a vegetable diet." Experiments on dogs and chickens failed to show any change in blood serum amylase regardless of whether a meat diet or carbohydrate diet was used, and Carlson determined also that the carnivorous dog and cat have a greater concentration of blood serum amylase than the herbivorous goat, sheep, ox, and rabbit. Serum amylase concentration has been found to be 10 to 12 times greater in the dog than in man: Schlesinger (35), Moeckel and Rost (36), Myers and Reid (37); and twice as great in the rabbit as in man: Watanabe (38), Schlesinger (35). The above references may be accepted as proof that food can cause no great variation in serum amylase, particularly not a variation of such magnitude as food can create in the digestive secretions or as exists in the several animal species. There are, however, a few reports showing that food does cause a mild and transient increase in the blood serum enzymes.

While the concentration of blood serum enzymes does not seem to be greatly influenced by food, it appears that digestive enzymes secreted into the fasting intestine can be detected in the blood. In his experiments on dogs, Boldyreff (18,39) showed that the muscles and glands comprising the digestive system are not at rest between the digestive acts. Juices are poured out and periodic rhythmic contractions occur in the digestive tube. These juices are absorbed and Boldyreff claims that at this time the protease and lipase content of the blood is increased. Ivanov and Basilewitsch (40) confirmed the conclusions of Boldyreff. Blood was examined during an experimental period when the contractions of the empty stomach were recorded, and it was found that blood lipase and amylase exhibited variations in amounts paralleling to a considerable degree the periodic activity of the digestive tract. It would be necessary, however, to rule out the possibility of these enzymes coming directly from the pancreas, liver, and other tissues, into the blood.

It is becoming generally recognized that the most effective stimulus to secretion of a particular enzyme is the type of food. As an example, amylase is secreted more abundantly in the presence of starch than when protein alone is the stimulating agent. Since the serum enzymes are not responsive to such alterations in the enzyme content of the intestine, it is plain they cannot be directly correlated with the digestive enzymes of the intestine. In view of these facts, it seems illogical to consider as competent any experiment designed to suggest the manner of disposition of intestinal digestive enzymes through tests upon the blood serum.

If further proof were needed that the absorption of digestive enzymes in large quantities is a normal physiological process, I could cite the fact that of the comparatively enormous quantities of enzymes poured into the gastrointestinal tube from the salivary glands, stomach, pancreas, and intestinal glands, only a small fraction can be recovered in the feces. That the enzymes are not inactivated by the feces, I have proved by liquefying the feces and allowing it to remain at 37 degrees C. for 24 hours. There was only a slight loss of activity in some of the experiments, while in others there seemed to be a slight increase by this treatment.

Digestive enzymes are removed from the intestine either through excretion with the feces or by absorption into the organism. Since only a comparatively small portion of the secretion is thrown out with the feces, the balance can disappear only by being absorbed into the body. To give some idea as to the relative amylolytic power of feces and body fluids, per gram and mL respectively, I shall review some representative data. The pioneer in this type of research is Wohlgemuth (41). It will be seen that the value of the secreted saliva alone is several times that of feces when 24 hours specimens are compared. The weight of human feces on a mixed diet is given by Howell (42) as less than 200 grams daily, and the secretion of pancreatic juice as 500 to 800 mL in 24 hours. Even if one considers Howell's figures for pancreatic juice secretion too high and prefers to accept the figure of 296 mL submitted by Villaret and Justin-Besancon (43), still there is seen to exist an enormous difference between the fecal values and the pancreatic juice values for amylase. Wohlgemuth's figures follow:

	Amylase
HUMAN FECES	468 units per gram
HUMAN SALIVA	1125 to 5,000 units per mL
HUMAN PANCREATIC JUICE	12,000 to 40,000 units per mL

It is seen that there is a vast difference between the quantity of enzymes secreted with the pancreatic juice into the intestine and the quantity finally eliminated in the feces - a difference possibly from 50 to 100 times as great, in favor of pancreatic juice. Although there is no information available on the value of enzymes secreted into the intestinal juice, it is thought to be considerable. So that the enzyme value of saliva, gastric juice, pancreatic juice, and intestinal juice secreted into the gastrointestinal tract left to be absorbed and not removed in the feces, constitutes by far the larger part of the whole secretion.

Sampogna (44) found human saliva to have high amylase content compared with the feces. The urine amylase value was usually greater than that of feces.

Harrison and Lawrence (45) found the following values for normal diastase content:

BLOOD	3 to 10 units
URINE	6.7 to 33.3 units

The figures of different workers are not comparable since various techniques are in use.

In normal babies, Morabito (46) arrived at the following values:

BLOOD	5 to 10 units
URINE	12 to 26 units

Whenever reference is made to "blood", blood serum is meant.

Gerner (47) made 114 tests on the urine and 90 on the blood of 49 healthy persons and determined the following amylase values:

BLOOD   8.8 to 22.8 units
URINE   16   to 128 units

According to Gray and Somogyi (48), in the healthy human, urine contains from 2 to 6 times as much amylase as blood does.

Zucker and associates (49) have shown that pancreatic juice contains at least 50 times greater concentration of amylase than serum.

Engelhardt and Gertschuk (50) presented the following figures on human amylase values:

BLOOD   3.85
URINE   8.23
SALIVA   1975.00

It is brought out by the foregoing data that the amylase content of urine is usually several times that of blood; that the value for feces is somewhat less than urine, while pancreatic juice or saliva is incomparably higher in amylase content. The only way to account for the large quantity of secreted enzymes which fail to reach the feces is to grant that they *must be absorbed* into the organism. When the varied forms of evidence presented are considered together, this conclusion is inescapable.

Chapter 4

EFFECT OF NATURE OF FOOD
ON ENZYME SECRETION

The available data supplies ample evidence that enzymes secreted into the intestine are repeatedly absorbed and secreted, over and over again, save for that portion voided by urine and feces. The evidence here presented shows that not only are *digestive enzymes reabsorbed,* but other enzymes supplied by barley malt, fungi, and dried pancreas extract are also absorbed into the organism in large quantities. The main difference between resting barley and germinated or malted barley is that the enzymes of barley are greatly multiplied during the course of germination. Comparison of enzymes found in wheat, barley, carrot, cabbage, milk, or honey, with the same enzymes contained in the digestive secretions shows that they possess the same characteristics, except for minor variations in pH optima for maximum activity. There is thus no basis for assuming that the enzymes present in natural food materials cannot be absorbed in the same manner as regular digestive enzymes.

It is not difficult to understand, on the basis of much recorded evidence, how ingested food enzymes can carry some of the burden of digestion and metabolism which otherwise must be assumed solely by the enzymes of the organism. Granting that the enzymes ingested daily by an individual following an exclusively raw food diet would comprise only a small fraction of the enzymes secreted every day into the digestive canal, it is nevertheless true that when these small amounts of food enzymes are taken into the digestive system every day for months or years, the total value of the enzymes consumed far exceeds not only the enzyme value of secreted digestive juices but also the enzyme value of the whole organism. If ingested food enzymes do a certain amount of work, which I propose to prove as a fact, then there will be correspondingly *less work* for the enzymes of the organism to perform and, consequently, there will be a weaker stimulus for secretion of tissues enzymes.

As a result, fewer body enzymes will be poured out into the secretions, fewer of them sacrificed, and more *conserved* within the tissues. That it is highly desirable to conserve the enzyme content of the tissues is proved by abundant evidence relating to the *progressive enzyme decrease* of body tissues and fluids *with increasing age.* Not only does the enzyme content decrease with increasing age, but it decreases markedly in many diseases.

It might be conjectured that the enzyme content of secreted digestive fluids has no relation to the nature of the food stimulus. Such, however, is not the case. Pavlov long ago maintained that *enzymes are secreted in response to specific stimuli - and starch stimulates the secretion of amylase, protein of protease, and fat that of lipase.*

Neilson and Lewis (51), Physiology Dept., University of St. Louis, tested the specific secretory response in 25 human subjects. Increase in salivary amylase of 30 to 60 per cent and even up to 150 per cent followed a carbohydrate diet, whereas a protein diet resulted in a decrease of 10 to 15 per cent salivary amylase. Neilson and Terry (52) had previously found that in dogs a carbohydrate diet produced saliva with considerable amylase but a meat diet resulted in a pronounced decrease or an entire absence of amylase. The small amount of amylase ordinarily present in the saliva of dogs and cats was considered by Carlson as adventitious. Mendel and Underhill were unable to obtain any evidence of the specific adaptation of the salivary glands of the dog to diet, but Samytschkina (53) proved, on dogs with parotid fistulae, that 4 to 7 days after rich carbohydrate diet, amylase appears in the saliva, rapidly reaches a maximum, then diminishes and disappears about 20 days later. Ingestion of any type of food led to no immediate change in the amylase content of the dog's saliva.

Simon (54) showed that human beings on a carbohydrate diet have saliva more powerfully amylolytic than when on a mixed diet. Saliva was tested every hour and on a carbohydrate diet it maintained its high activity much longer than the saliva secreted during and after a mixed diet. On a protein diet, the amylolytic power was less than on a mixed diet.

It was established by Evans (55) that after a meal containing fat, protein, and carbohydrate, the amylase content of human saliva rises. The increase begins within 20 to 30 minutes, reaches its maximum after 2 or 3 hours, followed by a fall. If a regular meal is omitted, the salivary amylase does not make its usual rise. A meal of protein alone is without effect.

Piccaluga (56) found a meal of carbohydrates causes an increase in the amount of human urinary amylase. After 5 days of carbohydrate diet the amount of amylase is increased still more. Four days after suspension of diet, amylase dropped to slightly higher than normal value.

Goldstein (57) concluded that the digestive power of human pancreatic juice depends on the kind of food given. Content of lipase, trypsin, and amylase depends on food.

The enzymic power of glycerol extracts of the pancreas of carnivorous, omnivorous, and herbivorous animals was investigated by Koldayev (58). A correlation was established with the nature of the food. Trypsin was found stronger in dogs than pigs, and weakest in oxen. Amylase was strongest in pigs, followed by oxen, and least in dogs. The investigation in respect to lipase gave no definite results.

Romijn (59) noted that the pancreas of the pig digested 1 percent solutions of various starches about 5 times as rapidly as that of the dog.

Krzywanek and Schakir (60) examined the enzyme content of the feces of the horse, cow, sheep, goat, pig, and dog. Feces of carnivora and omnivora contained much trypsin and little diastase, whereas those of herbivora contained little trypsin but much diastase. Lipase was found especially concentrated in the feces of pigs.

These facts, and those to be presented subsequently on the blood and urine amylase content in various species, are worthy of serious study. Since carnivora have relatively high amylase content in blood serum and relatively low amylase content in the urine, as compared with the amylase content of pancreas or feces; while herbivora have a relatively low amylase content in the blood serum and a relatively high content in the urine, as compared with their pancreas or fecal content, it is evident that a far greater correlation exists between the pancreas or feces and urine than between the blood serum and urine.

Further positive proof on the adaptivity of the digestive secretions to the character of the food is furnished by workers at the Russian Institute of Physiology. Working with pancreatic juice obtained from a human subject with a fistula of the pancreatic duct, Vasyutochkin and Drobintzeva found the concentration of different enzymes to be dependent on the diet - lipase increased with a fat diet, amylase with a carbohydrate diet, and trypsin with a meat diet.

Abramson (61) confirmed that the enzyme content of the pancreatic secretion on a mixed diet or on a diet poor in protein but rich in milk and carbohydrates tends to adjust itself to the character of the diet.

The highly specific and adaptable reaction of the organism to introduction of foreign substances into the blood stream confirms the point I wish to make concerning the specific response of enzyme production to specific stimulation. The Abderhalden reaction consists in the secretion of specific enzymes to specific stimuli. The physiologist Abderhalden and his associates (62-71 incl.) have shown by numerous experiments that when foreign substances such as sucrose, lactose, fibrin globulin, euglobulin, pseudoglobulin, and serum albumin are administered parenterally or subcutaneously, distinctive enzymes are eliminated in the urine which are highly specific for the type of material introduced. Administration of sucrose leads to sucrase excretion; lactose to lactase excretion; the proteins lead to excretion of those proteases which will attack only the particular type of protein administered.

Molinar (72) measured the lipase content of feces and detected considerable increase after ingestion of oil. He believes the increased fat content stimulates secretion of lipase by the intestine.

It is a remarkable fact that the young of most, if not all animals, including man, have weak digestive fluids; particularly do they have low amylase content in the saliva. The suckling animal or infant does not need to secrete a great quantity of enzymes because milk, its first food, does not demand so many of them for its digestion as it has quite a complement of its own enzymes.

In experiments on dogs with Thiry-Vella fistulae, it was demonstrated by Andreev and Georgiewsky (73,74,75), Institute of Pathological Physiology, First University, Moscow, that the amylase content of intestinal juice is directly proportional to the amount of starch in the diet, being least on a meat diet and increasing with an increase in the carbohydrate content of the ingested food. There was always a latent period of several days. The change in the amylase content occurred, not simultaneously with change in the diet, but later. This delayed response, which has also been observed by Samytschkina (53) in dog saliva, does not occur in man.

It can be safely accepted as a general principle that the amylase, protease, or lipase content of digestive fluids is determined essentially by the quantity of starch, protein, or fat present in ingested food. Evidence is supplied by the literature that there are times when the normal organism secretes quantities of digestive fluids below average enzyme content. It is to be presumed that when foods are ingested which require no digestion, such as dextrose, the stimulus for enzyme secretion is lacking, though other components of digestive juice may flow into the digestive canal quite normally.

Chapter 5

EFFICACY OF FOOD ENZYMES IN DIGESTION

Since enzymes are normally a part of the food, it follows that *food enzymes* have been spontaneously *assisting* in digestion, if not in metabolism, in the era before man became acquainted with use of fire. Likewise, no one can deny that intracellular and extracellular food enzymes become active after food is chewed and conditions of temperature and moisture are suitable, and that these food enzymes become active and have already performed work before the subsequent entrance of the enzymes composing the digestive secretions. Thus, I believe, the role of food enzymes is conditioned by circumstances beyond control when raw, uncooked food is consumed.

Taking up this question, Mangold and Dubiski (76), Institute of Animal Physiology, Agriculture College, Berlin, made comparative experiments of digestion of ground cereals and pure starch in the crop of living fowls and in the thermostat. The contents of the crop of fowls fed pure starch showed no erosion of the starch grains because of the absence of amylase from the salivary and crop secretions of the fowl. But erosion was evident (yield of soluble carbohydrates, especially sugar) on feeding ground barley and is to be attributed to the effect of the amylase in the grain. The crop, 5 hours after feeding ground barley, showed about 8 per cent soluble carbohydrate and 5 per cent sugar. The part of food enzymes in the digestion of starch in the animal body is estimated at 5 to 10 per cent. It is pointed out by Mangold and Dubiski that food enzymes may also play a further part in digestion in the stomach and intestine, even in animals with an active saliva.

Schwarz and Teller (77) measured the amount of water absorbed during the sojourn of wheat grains in the crop of live fowls. The increase in weight of the wheat grains, due to swelling was:

11.43% in 4 hours
32.69% in 6 hours
36.71% in 8 hours

The crop emptied in 11 to 12 hours after 30 grams of grain were fed. The authors believed that the enzyme reactions which occurred were due to enzymes present in the grains, since the secretion of the mucosa contains neither amylolytic nor proteolytic enzymes.

The proteolytic enzymes of oats, barley, and vetch were demonstrated by Aron (78) to digest easily the proteins of milk and the various vegetable proteins. The end point in the digestion is reached in 6 hours. Aron considers that these vegetable enzymes aid pepsin and trypsin.

In autolyses of various vegetable food stuffs used for domestic animals with a view of ascertaining how far the enzymes contained in these foods may aid in the digestion of their own constituents in the body, Grimmer (79) found that the proteolytic enzymes of horse beans, vetch, barley, and oats were very active. Determinations were made of the total dissolved nitrogen, coagulable protein, albumoses, etc.

Boas (80) demonstrated that the oxidizing enzymes of bananas (catalase, oxidase, and peroxidase) which were used as a test meal, are reactivated in the secretions of the intestine and serve several useful purposes. Similarly, Matveev (81) recorded experiments on the influence of the oxidase, peroxidase, and catalase supplied by carrot juice upon the digestive processes. A decrease of activity of the enzymes occurred in the acid medium of the stomach, but in the alkaline secretions of the duodenum a further increased activity of the enzymes could be detected. It is proposed by Matveev that these oxidation enzymes, which are supplied in the raw vegetable diet, are to be regarded as staple supplements to the enzymes necessary in the digestive process.

That saliva cannot digest raw starch *in vitro* can be determined easily with the aid of a microscope and has been reported many times. Reichert (82) has summarized the literature on this subject. And yet it is quite obvious that raw starch is regularly digested in large quantity in the organism. The fattening of farm animals by feeding raw corn and raw potato offers persuasive proof that raw starch undergoes digestion and assimilation. Mangold (83) states that there is no amylolytic action in the crop of pigeons but very active starch digestion in the intestinal tract. Penetration of hen's digestive juice into plant cells, such as corn glutin cells, is very slight and digestion of the protein and starch awaits rupture of these cells by what he calls "plasmolysis."

Pozerski's (84) experiments lead him to state that pre-treatment of raw starch with dilute hydrochloric acid aids in its subsequent digestion.

Roseboom and Patton (85,86) have shown that dogs can digest and absorb large quantities of raw corn starch. Up to 75 grams was fed to dogs weighing about 35 pounds, and the feces was found entirely free of starch by the iodine test. It was concluded that this quantity was digested. When glucose excretion was studied in phloridzinized dogs fed raw corn starch, it was found that nearly quantitative digestion of the starch occurred.

That a raw food diet, because of the lack of gustatory qualities of cooked food, does not call forth an abundant secretion of digestive enzymes is proved in several ways. Attention must be directed to the fact that the secretions of digestive glands also serve the purpose of lubrication and dilution. The quantity of a secretion does not alone determine its digestive power. Dry foods may call forth a large quantity of comparatively weak digestive fluid. The cow secretes enormous quantities of inactive saliva, solely for purposes of dilution and lubrication. It is appreciated by clinicians that food properly cooked, flavored, and seasoned, stimulates a greater quantity of digestive enzyme secretion than, for instance, a meal of raw vegetables. Convalescents, in whom digestion is weak, are customarily given tasty, appetizing, cooked dishes, which, through the senses of taste and smell, produce maximum secretions of digestive fluids.

That heat-treated foods do cause a greater outpouring of enzymes into the digestive canal than do raw foods is illustrated by the work of Buddle (87). Quantitative determinations of trypsin and peptidase were carried out on stools passed in 24 hours by breast-fed and bottle-fed babies. The relative amount of trypsin of breast-fed babies was significantly, and the amount of peptidase, markedly, lower than in bottle-fed babies. I interpret this to suggest that pasteurized milk requires the participation of more digestive enzymes than raw milk, and, consequently, that a *raw diet tends to be economical in its use and disposition of digestive enzymes,* while a heat-treated diet causes more of them to be used up and excreted.

Chapter 6

PANCREAS HYPERTROPHY
AND HEAT-TREATED DIET

The fact that the pancreas of herbivorous animals, subsisting exclusively upon raw plant substances, is relatively very small, offers convincing testimony for the important part played by food enzymes in digestion of raw foods. Thus, while the pancreas of a human subject of 140 pounds weighs 85 to 90 grams (88), the pancreas of sheep weighing 85 pounds (89) weighs only 18.8 grams (90); that of 1005 pound cattle (89), only 308 grams (90) and of horses weighing 1200 pounds, only 330 grams (91). Or, calculated as a percentage of the body weight, the following figures are evolved:

	Body weight Grams	Pancreas weight as % of body weight
Sheep	38,505	0.0490
Cattle	455,265	0.0680
Horse	543,600	0.0603
Camel (92)	509,400	0.0556
Man	63,420	0.1400

If digestion in herbivora depended exclusively upon secreted digestive enzymes, these animals should properly be expected to display highly active salivary glands to assume some of the burden of digestion. But, on the contrary, the saliva of these herbivora, relatively speaking, contains no enzymes as is well known to physiologists, and cannot even partially relieve the pancreas of the duty of starch digestion, let alone help in protein and fat digestion. It must be considered as remarkable that animals living upon a diet consisting largely of carbohydrates should have inactive salivary glands and small pancreatic glands. What other explanation can be given than that the enzymes naturally present in food relieve the animal body of the work of digestion to a considerable extent. The facts standing out in bold relief are:

The raw food of herbivora supplies active enzymes which participate in diges-tion. Active salivary glands are not required and there is no need for a large pancreas. On the other hand, the diet of man is grossly deficient in food en-zymes, his salivary glands are highly active, and the human pancreas is pro-portionally at least twice as large··· as that of herbivora.

It might be brought out that the long intestine of herbivora sup-plies sufficient *succus entericus* to compensate for other secretions. How-ever, there is no good reason for assuming that because the intestine is long there will be a commensurate increase in its secretion. The expla-nation evidently does not hold true since the horse and rabbit have relatively short, small intestines for herbivorous animals and both also display relatively small pancreatic glands.

These facts suggest clearly that the *enzymes present in raw, uncooked food relieve the pancreas and salivary glands of the necessity of enlarging from excess work.* The considerable hypertrophy of the pancreas and salivary glands, which has been found to occur in human races living upon large quantities of cooked carbohydrates, indicates the nature of the intrepid but deplorable compensatory measures the organism is forced to adopt, and is added proof of the profound influence and ben-efit of enzymes supplied naturally by raw foods.

That the pancreas and salivary glands of human beings living upon the customary heat-treated enzyme-deficient diet are hypertrophied and overworked organs is not difficult to believe. Those races subsist-ing largely upon heat-treated carbohydrates appear to have the largest pancreatic and salivary glands. Thus, Sitsen (93,94) has shown that the pancreas of Malays of Java has an average weight of 105 grams, while the average weight of the American pancreas is about 20 grams less. And this in spite of the fact that Americans average some 20 or 30 pounds heavier in body weight than Javanese. Sitsen observed that other organs are heavier in occidentals than in Malays, excepting the pancreas and salivary glands which alone are heavier in Malays. He attributes the large pancreas and salivary glands of Malays to a diet rich in carbohydrates.

In an extensive study of the organ weights of adult Filipinos dying by violence or accident, DeLeon and associates (95), School of Hygiene and Public Health, University of the Philippines, subjected 768 such bodies to post-mortem examination over a period of years. This was an unusual study in that the subjects had been comparatively healthy. By comparing weights of the principal organs of Filipinos with those of occidentals as given by Jackson (96), DeLeon and co-workers were able to confirm the observations of Sitsen. They found that the visceral organs of Europeans and Americans were on the whole heavier than the same organs of Filipinos, with the exception of the pancreas, which was heavier in Filipinos. Salivary glands were not studied. The figures on Filipinos are:

Number of Cases	Sex	Pancreas Wt. Grams	Body weight Pounds	Pancreas weight as % of body wt.
121	M	105.9	106	0.22
39	F	86.2	90	0.21

On Americans, the only extensive investigation recorded on the weight of the pancreas was by Schaefer (97), Mayo Foundation and University of Minnesota. Although this study was not confined to persons dying by violence or accident, it is considered by Schaefer to indicate the average normal weight of the pancreas, since no organs with extensive pathological changes were included. Schaefer's figures, based on 216 personally collected cases, follow:

MALE	90.31 grams,	plus or minus 15.08
FEMALE	84.88 grams,	plus or minus 14.95

Assuming as a conservative estimate that the average body weight of Americans is only 20 to 40 pounds more than the average weight of the adult Filipino, the following calculation can be arranged:

Body weight Pounds	Pancreas wt. Grams (aver. Of m. & f.)	Pancreas wt as % of body wt.
120	87.6	0.16
130	87.6	0.15
140	87.6	0.14

The foregoing data brings out the important fact that the pancreas of Filipinos and Malays is both relatively and absolutely heavier than that of occidentals; relatively about 25 to 50 per cent heavier. When it is recalled that cooked rice is the staple article of food among Filipinos, commonly eaten three times each day, the reason for the extra pancreas tissue can be comprehended. The food of Americans contains less carbohydrate and more protein, and while it may not be considered to be less denatured by heat than Filipino food, the burden for its digestion is shared by the stomach, and in this circumstance probably resides the explanation as to the reason for the unusual pancreatic hypertrophy among races using large amounts of heat-treated carbohydrate food.

Mikulicz's disease is considered to be a compensatory hypertrophy of the parotid glands, responding to a failing pancreas. John (98) reported 4 cases of chronic parotid enlargement, all of whom were mild diabetics and obese.

Flaum (99,100) investigated 27 cases of Mikulicz's disease and claimed it is of frequent occurrence in diabetes. There was a more or less marked glycosuria on an ordinary diet in 16 cases. The 11 cases without glycosuria, when submitted to sugar tolerance tests, showed a failing sugar tolerance.

Glaser and Bannet (101) accounted for the hypertrophy of the salivary glands observed in diabetes by the observation that the salivary secretion supplements the activity of the pancreas. Chemical analysis of the salivary glands failed to reveal the presence of insulin.

Additional cases of Mikulicz's syndrome are reported by Charvat [year 1932] and Dobreff [year 1936]. Since many experimental undertakings have failed to show that the salivary glands are capable of supplying an insulin-like internal secretion, the phenomena attending Mikulicz's disease can only be interpreted as being a compensatory over-production of salivary enzymes to assume some of the burden of carbohydrate metabolism.

Pursuing farther the contention that *heat-denatured, enzyme-deficient food places unnatural strain upon the enzyme secreting organs,* I can show that changes in the weight of the pancreas and other organs have been repeatedly induced experimentally in animals by use of such diets. Jackson (102), Dept. of Anatomy, University of Minnesota, has shown statistically the weight changes in organs of rats who were fed for a period of about 155 days on a diet, properly balanced for salts and vitamins, comprising 80 per cent heat-treated carbohydrate. The pancreas and submaxillary glands increased in weight 20 to 30 per cent. The pituitary and suprarenals decreased in weight. The organs were carefully dissected and weighed, using a uniform technique.

The question arises, why should the pancreas and salivary gland increase in weight under the influence of a heat-treated, carbohydrate diet if the increased capacity is not sponsored by a need for more digestive enzymes. It is an inescapable conclusion that on a heat-treated carbohydrate diet the pancreas is called upon to supply more enzymes than where the diet consists of both carbohydrate and protein. To appraise the status of the enzymes naturally supplied in food, it is only necessary to remember that, whereas a heat-treated enzyme-deficient carbohydrate diet induces pancreatic hypertrophy in human races and experimental animals, a raw, uncooked carbohydrate diet, containing its natural enzymes, contributes to a relatively small pancreas and inactive salivary glands in the herbivora. At first thought, it might be presumed that hypertrophy of the pancreas is a desirable accommodation. But there is always the tendency for the hypertrophy of excessive function to proceed to the atrophy of exhaustion. An atrophy of the pancreas occurs in many terminal wasting diseases. In avitaminosis experiments, there is always a primary hypertrophy of the pancreas followed by a terminal atrophy. Furthermore, the elaborate investigations and organ weight measurements of Brown, Pearce and Van Allen (103,104,105) of Rockefeller Institute for Medical Research prove it is impossible for one organ to change in weight without promoting compensatory weight alterations in all organs. This need not be considered remarkable when the interactions of hormones, enzymes and vitamins are taken into account. The vast influence on bodily functions of such profound anatomical modifications should be recognized as the precursor of symptomatic developments.

Under the circumstances, and in view of the facts that have been uncovered, I believe it to be the solemn duty of all interested in the advancement of science to apply themselves diligently to making these principles more generally known so that the possible influence of *food enzymes* upon human *welfare* can be fully appreciated.

Chapter 7

ENZYME CONTENT OF BODY
FLUIDS IN DISEASE

It may be asserted that the enzymes naturally present in foods are not necessary to human health and the digestive secretions contain enough enzymes to digest all foods. What proof can be submitted that such statements are based on fact? The important question is not whether the digestive secretions contain sufficient enzymes during one meal or during any limited time, but rather whether it is compatible with *extended good health and a life span of reasonable duration* to sanction the daily depreciation occurring when rich concentrations of secreted enzymes are poured into the gastrointestinal canal in response to excess stimulation from heat-treated food.

Statements that saliva is efficient in itself and not dependent upon the enzymes of foods is true, with reservations. *Similarly, it may be observed that a drunkard, with his weekly wage in his pocket, can display the semblance of prosperity and competency for a day.* In recent years, we have witnessed how nations can maintain an appearance of solvency and prosperity by borrowing against future resources. I believe the question confronting those interested in health conservation is not whether saliva or other digestive fluids have the capacity to digest all foods, but rather whether it is in the interest of *optimum health* and *longer life* to allow the unaided digestive fluids to perform this work for extended periods of time.

It is a fact, which I will elucidate and for which sufficient proof will be submitted, that the enzyme-producing power, or the *enzyme reserve* of the organism, is fixed within definite *limits*. The speed of metabolism is determined by the quantity of enzymes engaged. The greater the metabolic exchange within the tissues, the more enzymes are required to participate and, consequently, the greater will be the quantity of them wasted by excretion.

Dehlhougne (106) examined the blood of 20 normal human subjects for catalase, protease, peroxidase, and esterase and found a marked increase under the influence of physical work. Gerner (107) made 3,000 amylase determinations on the blood and urine in 115 patients, representing 28 different acute infectious diseases. The urinary amylase was increased in 73 per cent of the cases examined; the blood amylase in 38 per cent.

Kreyberg (108) found increased elimination of amylase in the urine in several acute febrile diseases, as compared to a normal value obtained from the urine of 235 persons. Pavel and associates (109) noted increased amylase content in the blood and urine of 18 cases of pneumonia. The amylase content of the blood and urine ran parallel. Thomasen (110) observed increased amylase output in the urine in patients with acute appendicitis.

The peptidase content of the serum in paresis is normal, according to Pfeiffer (111). If a paretic is infected with malaria, the serum peptidase rises to 10 to 20 times the former value. Other febrile conditions, such as erysipelas and advanced pulmonary tuberculosis, also increase the peptolytic index of the serum. The peptidases of the serum rise with the fever.

In relapsing fever, Solovtzova (112) found the proportion of proteolytic enzymes in the urine generally increased at the crisis. The amount of amino acids in the urine gradually increases beginning with the attack and through to the crisis, when it jumps suddenly still higher. Lipase generally increase toward the crisis. The most important cause of the favorable or unfavorable course and issue of infectious disease in man, according to Solovtzova, is the condition of the relation between the enzymes of the organism and the degree of affinity between them and the infecting agent.

Spinelli (113) rendered guinea pigs hyperthermic by injection of an autolyzate of beer yeast. While the fever was at its maximum, the animals were killed and the time of reduction of m-dinitrobenzene by various tissues was measured. There was an increased power of reduction in the hyperthermic animals, indicating increased dehydrogenase content. A similar increase was found when the oxidase was tested.

Frohlich and Neumann (114), using human substratum isolated from normal lung and kidney, tested proteolysis with 54 serums from tubercular and non-tubercular patients. Proteolysis of 5.0 mg per cent was normal for the lung and 2.7 per cent for the kidney. In cases of pulmonary tuberculosis, the proteolysis may vary from 21 mg per cent to 0.0 mg per cent. The low values occur in afebrile cases with gain of weight and the high values in febrile cases with loss of weight. Pneumonia, lung infarcts, and other non-tuberculous lung processes display increased protease content of the serum. In these diseases, according to Frohlich and Neumann, the protease content of the serum is a measure of the defensive power of the organ involved.

In a carefully conducted and long continued investigation of the urinary amylase output, Eckhardt (115), City Pediatric Clinic, Essen, Germany, found high values to be characteristic of high fevers in children. He (116) found high urinary values for amylase in pregnancy and pneumonia. According to the findings of Bach and Lustig (117), cadaver blood serum showed a very marked increase in lipolytic action in acute feverish diseases.

Ma (118) found the peptidase content of serum and urine of children in infectious diseases and fevers to be increased. The peptidase content of blood and urine gave a definite curve for each febrile disease studied by Bohmig (119). In pneumonia, peptidase was shown to rise abruptly at the crisis and soon after fall to normal, accompanied by an increased excretion in the urine.

Increase in metabolic activity, whether associated with fever, accelerated heart action, increased food intake, muscular work, or pregnancy, is paralleled by rise in the enzyme content of the blood and increased enzyme loss in the urine. In febrile conditions, metabolism is speeded up and enzyme activity is likewise increased, as the above reports show. It is interesting to note that one of the main characteristics of all enzymes is their accelerated activity with rising temperature. In other words, enzymes are more active, and will perform more work, in the organism as well as *in vitro*, at a fever temperature of 104°F than at the normal body temperature. This illustrates the precision with which coordination operates within the organism. There is *much evi-*

dence to indicate that the response of enzymes to elevation in temperature functions as the main mechanism in defense of the body against bacteria and other invading agents. Bearing on this point, Solaroli (120) found that in experimental hyperthermia and in human fever, the blood catalase activity increases during the increase of temperature and suffers sudden drop when the temperature falls.

At normal body temperature, however, the blood content of catalase has been shown to be correlated with the degree of metabolism (121). Exposure to cold (winter) decreases the metabolism of cold-blooded animals and decreases the metabolism of pine needles (122); the catalase content is likewise proportionally decreased in both instances. On the other hand, summer temperatures exert reverse effects on the metabolism and catalase content. In the case of warm-blooded animals, measurements by Burge (122) indicate that both metabolism and blood catalase content are increased in cold weather and decreased in summer. Viale (123) likewise found that the amount of catalase in the blood increases as the temperature decreases at normal body temperature.

The quickened metabolism and oxidation after ingestion of food is associated with heightened catalase content of the blood according to the researches of Burge and Neill (124), and Burge and Leichsenring (124a), University of Illinois. These workers believe oxidation, following ingestion of food, especially food of high calorie value, such as meat and fat, is attributable to increase in catalase produced by stimulation of the digestive glands, particularly the liver. Starvation caused decrease in blood catalase.

It is well known that during the accelerated activity associated with germination of seeds, the content of various enzymes markedly increases. Pett (125), Biochemical Institute, University of Stockholm, measured the amounts of dipeptidase, protease and lipase in dormant and germinating wheat seeds and observed a variable increase in these enzymes after germination.

Phosphatase activity in beans (126), potatoes, radishes, and wheat was determined by Wasteneys, Dept. of Biochemistry, University of

Toronto, during dormancy, germination, and maturation. The greatest phosphatase content was during the period of greatest activity - germination. During the period of maturation, enzyme activity fell.

Swanson (127) compared the amylase activity of germinated whole wheat grains, germinated germ ends, and germinated brush ends, and found a great increase in activity in all parts when compared with dormant seeds. Many studies are recorded confirming the rise in amylase activity corresponding with the increased metabolism of germinating wheat and barley grains. Jono (128) tested the seed and seedlings of six common plants for amylase, maltase, pepsin, trypsin, erepsin, lipase, urease, catalase, and nuclease. Where the enzymes were present in the seed, their activity usually increased during the germinating, seedling stage.

During the increased metabolism of pregnancy, Vercesi (129) observed a steady increase in blood and urine amylase content. Katsu (130) found serum of puerperal women contained a large amount of catalase.

Ammon and Schutte (131) isolated the esterases, tributyrinase, cholinesterase, and methylbutyrase in the hen's egg and found that these enzymes undergo hardly any quantitative alteration during the first 5 days of incubation, but from then on their amount increases rapidly. Similar determinations were made on dipeptidases.

Koebner (132) found human and animal saliva contained a lipase. In 20 cases in human pregnancy, salivary lipase increased up to the time of delivery and the value also remained above normal during lactation.

Hileman and Courtney (133) stated that the amount of lipase in cows' milk produced in New York is at a minimum in June or July and at a maximum in December or January, and that one of the factors governing lipase secretion is the lactation cycle, the amount increasing with advancing lactation.

Various investigators (134,135,130,136) have reported that colostrum contains increased quantities of amylase and catalase which rapidly diminish after delivery.

Proof is supplied in the foregoing pages that carbohydrates, fats, and proteins exert specific stimulation for secretion of the corresponding enzymes. Manifestly, if part of the ingested food is digested by its own enzymes, the stimulus for secretion of the particular enzyme will be correspondingly weakened, with the result that less of it will be secreted and more of it retained within the tissues. In other words, the facts indicated that starch stimulates secretion of amylase; protein, protease; and fat, lipase. If a certain percentage, say 5, 10, or 20 per cent of the starch, protein, or fat is digested by food enzymes and changed into substances which do not require further digestion and therefore do not stimulate secretion of any type of enzyme, that percentage of 5, 10, or 20 does not need enzymes from the tissues which will ordinarily be required when food enzymes are not at hand to assist with digestion. Consequently, it may be said to be very desirable to allow *food enzymes to perform as much of the wok of digestion as possible in the interest of conserving the enzyme potential of the tissues.* When the food is so prepared and served that it lacks enzymes, the substitution of other suitable enzymes is in line with the trend of the evidence.

Chapter 8

NUTRITIONAL ROLE OF EXOGENOUS ENZYMES

I believe that the facts enumerated in these pages permit one to take the position that food enzymes are biologically normal and necessary if there is to be a full measure of health and a life span of reasonable duration. However, it may also be asserted that the food enzymes are not necessary for good health; that the digestive glands can produce all of the necessary digestive enzymes and that the body tissues can produce the enzymes required for metabolism. But the facts at hand make this position untenable, and I propose to prove it is not sound.

In the first place, practically all human beings ingest food enzymes every day. A small quantity of raw food is used by nearly everyone. It cannot be denied, therefore, that food enzymes do a tangible, though variable, quantity of work in all average persons. Since all enzymes are extremely active substances, requiring only suitable conditions of temperature and moisture for optimum activity, it is reasonable to assume that food enzymes become active and have already performed work before the digestive enzymes are secreted in any great quantities and mixed with the food. This point can be very conveniently proved in the chicken, pigeon, and those herbivora with inactive salivary glands. Secondly, bacteria swallowed with food, water, and air, contain enzymes. While neither the quantity of bacteria ingested nor the quantity finally finding a suitable abode in the intestine may be large, the number of them developing, after a few hours, in the warm, moist intestine is known to be enormous. A considerable part of the feces has been stated by Kendall (137), Northwestern University, to be composed of the bodies of bacteria. Using the food of the host as a culture medium, the quantity of enzymes produced by these countless bacteria must be considerable and they are placed at the selective disposal of the organism. It cannot be denied that bacteria are efficient and prolific enzyme producers since highly active bacterial enzymes are being used regularly in industry. The fact that bacterial action takes place principally in the colon is not poignant since it has been established that periodically occurring reversal of peristalsis is perhaps a normal condition in the intestinal tract.

Thus the *argument that the human race seems to get along satisfactorily without the help of accessory enzymes is not valid.* However, the propriety of depending upon enzymes from bacterial sources is open to question, and I have evidence indicating that the unnatural appropriativeness of enzyme-deficient organisms for bacterial enzymes engenders susceptibility to bacterial diseases.

It may, therefore, be concluded from the above that human beings are regularly receiving supplies of accessory enzymes. But what of the animals? Can they also live and remain in good health without them? A large scale feeding experiment has been conducted for the past five years upon dogs by Swift & Co., makers of a canned dog food. The dogs receive nothing but the canned food and water and it has been reported that reproduction, appetite, condition of hair, and general health have not suffered. Since the dogs get no food besides the canned product, which has been rendered enzyme-free by heat sterilization, it might be argued that here is proof that the animal organism can do without accessory enzymes. Before coming to such a conclusion, however, an analysis of all facts pertaining to the problem is warranted.

At a suitable temperature, bacteria, molds, and yeasts naturally present in the air can rapidly effect profound changes in various liquid materials, such as milk and grape juice. Laboratory experience teaches the immense propensity for rapid reproduction of these low forms of life. Not only do the dogs receive an unlimited supply of bacteria, molds, and yeasts directly from the air, but the moist food, while in the feeding trough, accumulates these organisms and offers a congenial culture medium. After being eaten and transported to the intestine, the food is again subjected to attack by a teeming bacterial population which vies for it with the secreted enzymes, with the result that the animal is actually furnished with no small quantity of accessory enzymes. That bacterial life in the intestine is prolific and may furnish considerable quantities of accessory enzymes to the organism may be surmised from the investigations of Kendall (137), Northwestern University Medical School, who concluded that about 50 per cent of the total nitrogen of the feces is contained in the bodies of dead bacteria. These experiments of Swift & Co. which have been widely advertised in magazines, cannot, therefore, be interpreted as substantiating the contention that animals can maintain good health without the aid of accessory enzymes. Furthermore, not even the oldest of the animals have yet passed the period of middle age, and it remains to be seen whether they will fare any better in latter life than rats fed purified but balanced diets. It is doubtful if this experiment can be used as a criterion of the sufficiency of a cooked diet since it has not been published and it is not possible to obtain much important information bearing upon it. This particular food contains a surplus of vitamins A, B, D, and G to compensate for amounts destroyed during the cooking and sterilizing operations.

Since it is impossible to eliminate the influence of bacterial accessory enzymes in the ordinary experiment, it becomes extremely important, in order to evaluate the status of food enzymes in normal nutrition and metabolism, to learn the condition of health of animals reared under asceptic conditions, given sterile food with the usual sterile vitamin accessories, and allowed to drink only sterile water and breathe only sterile air. Just such an experiment has been in progress at the Laboratories of Bacteriology, University of Notre Dame, for the past 12 years, during which time more than 2,000 germ-free guinea pigs, as well as germ-free chicks, rats, mice, rabbits, cats, and insects were born and reared under rigidly asceptic conditions. Dr. Reyniers, who conducts the work, has designed much special apparatus to enable the technique to be more easily carried out. The original purpose of the experiments was to establish and perfect a procedure whereby sterile laboratory animals would be available for the use of bacteriologists. Animals are delivered by Cesarean section under such conditions that the intestinal tract remains sterile. They are then allowed to breathe only sterile air and eat and drink only germ-free food and water.

Every day a bacteriological test is made of every accessible body cavity. Directly after birth, one of the litter is sacrificed and its body reduced to pulp by grinding. A suitable amount of this pulp is incubated with 22 different kinds of culture media. Sterility of the intestinal tract during the lifetime of the animal is assured by frequent tests for bacteria. Reyniers' sterile animals often grow to unusual size, but very few of them are healthy. It is stated that their digestive tracts are "delicate" and they apparently lack something which germs could furnish them. In a personal communication, Dr. Reyniers stated that sterile animals are on the whole a little more susceptible to infectious diseases than animals raised normally, and that a great many organic diseases show up in germ-free animals. He further stated that all foods used are exposed to a temperature of $250^{O}F$ for periods of 20 minutes to one hour. Vitamin loss is made up through use of sterile concentrates. Under these conditions the animals are deprived *only* of all accessory *enzymes. It is evident, therefore, that symptoms of impaired health in germ-free animals cannot be ascribed to vitamin deficiency,* since special care was used to counterbalance any such shortfall. Furthermore, the fact that they have a tendency to grow beyond normal size seems more than to fulfill the tenets of the vitamin philosophy and speaks in favor of vitamin sufficiency.

It is thus apparent that when the conditions of experiment are such as to eliminate the possibility of any accessory enzymes reaching the intestine, the health of the animal organism suffers. This is strong indication that *food enzymes* are *indispensable* for normal health and a life span of moderate duration.

The possibility exists that bacteria may favorably influence the health of a host in some other way than by acting as agents for manufacture of enzymes. This possibility is rendered less likely, however, when it is considered that the intestinal tract of the newly-hatched chick and the intestinal tracts and feces of the young of animals and man (137) are sterile at birth. It is made still more unlikely and difficult of acceptance when it is pointed out that the intestinal tracts of white bears, seal, reindeer, eider ducks, and penguins were found by Levin (138), to be sterile in the animals living in the Arctic regions. But when these same animals and birds are brought to a temperate climate, Corson-White (139) found they acquire bacteria rapidly. The fact that mammals and birds living in the Arctic regions can live normally on their natural, uncooked diet, under adverse environmental conditions, without intestinal bacteria, coupled with the fact that experimental animals, kept free of bacteria and fed with an enzyme-free diet, develop impaired health, makes it virtually certain that the indispensableness of bacteria to a host living upon a heat-treated diet consists mainly in a legacy of bacterial accessory enzymes.

Since animal inhabitants of Arctic regions preserve normal health without intestinal bacteria on a diet containing the natural quota of food enzymes, and since experimental animals kept free of intestinal bacteria cannot maintain normal health on a diet totally lacking in food enzymes, the conclusion that the only factor responsible for the difference in the health standards of the two groups is the *presence* of *food enzymes* in the diet of one group and their absence in the diet of the other, becomes irrefutable.

Chapter 9

ENZYMES OF BLOOD SERUM AND URINE IN ANIMALS

A fact which has much bearing upon the matter under discussion relates to the comparatively low amylase content of human blood serum as compared with that of domestic animals.

Reid and Myers (140) gave the following average values for blood serum amylase, using the sugar reduction method:

MAN	16
RABBIT	30
DOG	175

Schlesinger (141) arrived at the following comparative averages, using the Wohlgemuth method:

MAN	15 (10 TO 20)
RABBIT	29 (25 TO 33)
OX	39 (38 TO 40)
DOG	210 (170 TO 250)

Moeckel and Rost (142), using a sugar reduction method, placed man lowest among animals in the scale of blood serum amylase content; yet the amount of enzyme lost in the urine was comparable to that of other animals:

	Blood	*Urine*
MAN	6	40
RABBIT	9	45
SHEEP	11	12
GOAT	14	?
OX	17	?
CAT	44	30

GUINEA PIG	45	54
DOG	80	36
SWINE	103	55
RAT	?	65

King's (143) researches at the University of Chicago, disclosed that man ranks high in the amount of amylase eliminated in urine. Unfortunately no figures were supplied for human blood serum (Wohlgemuth method):

	Blood	Urine
MAN	?	1.53
GOAT	0.53	0.013
RABBIT	2.50	1.05
DOG	6.20	0.12
PIG	6.60	1.46
CAT	6.80	0.33
WOODCHUCK	18.00	9.00
RACCOON	20.00	0.34

Using a sugar reduction method, LoMonaco (144), Institute of Biological Chemistry, Palermo, established the following values for amylase content in different species:

	Blood	Urine
OX	7.1	3.1
RABBIT	8.2	9.0
CHICKEN	9.8	?
DOG	18.8	6.2
PIG	31.4	6.0

Wohlgemuth (145) arrived at the following average figures for blood amylase in an extensive study with the method bearing his name:

OX	22
GOAT	32
RABBIT	55
DOG	250
GUINEA PIG	521

Wohlgemuth (146) found man excretes more amylase than the dog or rabbit.

A study of the foregoing figures discloses the remarkable fact that human blood serum displays relatively the smallest amount of amylase of any of the animals tested. Another important point revealed by these findings is that the amount of amylase lost in human urine is totally out of proportion to the amount present in human blood serum. The concentration of amylase in human urine is shown to compare approximately with that of animal urines, while the blood content is disproportionately low. The explanation for this *apparent paradox must reside in the fact that man is the only animal whose diet is so extensively subjected to the destructive effects of cookery and pasteurization.* Thereby, a preponderantly large portion of its enzymes is destroyed, resulting in a failure of the organism to receive these enzymes and the necessity, consequently, of a secretion of them from the tissues in greater than physiologic amounts. Because more of them are secreted, more of them will be wasted and finally thrown out in the urine. Since this evidence correlates nicely with other valuable evidence previously cited, I cannot think of a reason why any other explanation should be sought.

Chapter 10

pH OF ENDOGENOUS AND
EXOGENOUS ENZYMES

There are no essential differences in characteristics between tissue enzymes and those consumed with food. The optimum pH for activity of food enzymes has a wide range, depending upon the type of enzyme and the substrate upon which it is tested. Likewise the enzymes found in animal organisms have a wide range of activity. There is no reason to assume that the enzymes ingested in food could not be adapted to the exact requirements of the organism. It should be no more difficult for the animal organism to convert vegetable or other food enzymes into animal enzymes (assuming that conversion is necessary) than it is for it to change vegetable protein into animal protein, or vegetable starch into animal glycogen.

That the pH characteristics of enzymes can be modified by the chemistry of the organism is suggested by certain experimental observations. Northrop's (147) experiments throw light on the mechanism by which certain characteristics of enzymes may become changed by keeping them in solutions of varying hydrogen-ion concentration (i.e. varying pH). Willstatter (148) described how the pH characteristics of enzymes may be modified: "Strong HCl or even better, pepsin in acid medium, causes a remarkable change in the nature of castor-bean lipase. After such treatment it coincides in its properties with the lipase of the germinating bean. The lipase of the dormant bean and the lipase of the germinating bean, behave like two entirely different enzymes. The one acts in acid medium, the other at neutrality."

It is well established that the optimum pH for enzymes varies with the temperature. For instance, Compton (149) showed that maltase at 47°C functions best at pH 7.2, while at a temperature of 35.5°C its maximum activity is at pH 3.0. More data on these points will be found in subsequent pages. The following table shows that the characteristics of endogenous and exogenous enzymes, referring to the organism, are similar.

Optimum pH of endogenous enzymes Of the animal organism			*Optimum pH of exogenous enzymes*		
Amylase, human saliva	(150)	6.0	Amylase, barley malt	(152)	4.4
Amylase, cattle saliva	(151)	6.5-6.6	Amylase, potato	(153)	6.7
Amylase, horse saliva	(151)	6.2	Amylase, cabbage	(154)	6.0
Amylase, pancreas	(152)	7.0	Amylase, carrot	(154)	6.0
			Amylase, white turnip	(154)	6.0
			Amylase, asper. oryzae	(152)	4.8
			Amylase, barley	(155)	4.5-4.7
			Amylase, wheat	(156)	4.6
			Amylase, rice malt	(157)	4.6
			Amylase, maize	(158)	5.0
			Amylase, sweet potato	(159)	5.5-6.0
			Amylase, banana	(160)	6.4
			Amylase, honey	(161)	5.3
			Amylase, cow's milk	(162)	6.3-6.7

Protease, pancreas	(163-4-5)	5.5-8.3	Protease, soy bean	(173)	4-8
Protease, gastric	(166-7)	1.2-1.8	Protease, yeast	(174)	4-4.5
Protease, intestine	(168)	7.7	Protease, yeast	(175)	6.8-8.5
Protease, human saliva	(169)	8.0	Protease, papaya	(176)	5.0
Protease, lymph glands	(170)	4.0	Protease, asper.oryzae	(177)	5.1
Protease, leukocyte	(171)	4.0	Protease, wheat malt	(178)	4.1
Protease,spleen, liver & kidney	(172)	4.5			

Lipase, human saliva	(179)	7.0	Lipase, asper.flavus	(187)	5.0
Lipase, human saliva	(180)	7.5-7.7	Lipase, wheat	(188)	7.3-8.2
Lipase, dog saliva	(181)	7.6-7.8	Lipase, takadiastase	(189)	8.6
Lipase, tortoise saliva	(182)	8.2	Lipase, castor bean	(190)	4.7-5.6
Lipase, pancreas	(183)	8.3-8.9			
Lipase, blood serum	(183)	8.0			
Lipase, stomach	(184)	6.0			
Lipase, tonsil	(185)	7.8-8.4			
Lipase, liver	(186)	6.7-8.2			

Catalase, liver	(191)	7.0	Catalase, vegetable	(154)	7-10
Catalase, leukocyte	(192)	7.0	Catalase, barley malt	(193)	7-8

Organs and tissues exhibit two optima for maximum activity. The greatest proteolysis occurs at pH 4 to 5 but there is also a smaller proteolysis at pH 7 to 8. At pH 4 to 5, cathepsin is active while at 7 to 8, tissue trypsin is active.

Chapter 11

VITAL COMPONENT OF THE
ENZYME COMPLEX

To account for all the facts and get a clearer conception of the manner the organism modifies the characteristics of *enzymes*, it is necessary to look upon enzymes not merely as catalysts, but as autocatalysts - particles of matter charged with what Professor Moore (194), University of Oxford, called, "*biotic energy*." Moore, in a detailed presentation, shows clearly the distinction between enzymes and metallic catalysts. Catalysts are not vital substances; enzymes are. According to Moore: "Living matter is inhabited by a type of energy bound to living matter and not producible in its absence. Enzymes appear to possess properties intermediate between dead colloids and living cells and carry outside of the cell certain properties belonging to living matter. Biochemistry may be defined as the study of the chemical substances produced by biotic energy - that is the energy of life - in the bodies of living plants and animals, and the further study of the energy processes by which such substances are elaborated and used subsequently to their production for carrying on the life of the cell. Enzymes differ from inorganic catalysts in that they are colloids, and to this, certain of the differences in action between inorganic catalysts and enzymes are due."

Establishment of enzymes as chemical substances has failed because of an improper perspective of their nature. Study of the biological as well as chemical facts relating to the characteristics of enzymes, evolves such a strong consensus of opinion that it becomes mandatory to consider enzymes vital substances - matter impregnated with energy values. At first thought, this might suggest a departure from the sphere of science to that of philosophy. But I fail to see why it should be more difficult to form such a conception of enzymes than it is to conceive of a flashlight battery as possessed of energy. In neither case is it necessary to leave anything to assumption since the energy values may be measured in both instances. *When a battery is "dead", the energy value has vanished; similarly, when enzymes are destroyed by heat, the energy value disappears, leaving behind only its vehicle.*

This concept of enzymes is by no means novel or original with me. A clear exposition of the idea is provided by Troland (195), Harvard University, in the following words: "The conception which, in my belief, constitutes the secret of life, is the conception of catalysis. There are, of course, many other processes in living organisms besides catalysis, but it is my thesis that the peculiarly vital properties of living beings depend directly upon catalytic action, or upon the developmental history of catalytic systems. The essence of life is catalysis, and this is no vitalistic 'entelechy', but a plain physico-chemical process. *Life*, according to this conception, is something which has been built up about the enzyme; it is a corollary of *enzyme activity*".

In a thought-provoking, critical review, involving 250 references to the literature, Ekman (196) places much emphasis on the autocatalytic theory of life. Life is regarded as a special form of autocatalysis, and organisms as fundamentally, autocatalysts. The essential nature of autocatalysts does not lie in their ability to catalyze reactions.

Laird (197), University of Iowa, presented an illuminating discussion on the true nature of enzymes. Quoting him: "While the functioning of living cells is dependent on their electrolytic as well as their colloidal structure, and both the inorganic components are essential, nevertheless, the dynamic, driving power, which apparently introduces the '*spark of life*', is found in their *enzymic contents*. The metaphysical entelectical explanations of life are scarcely needed since the discovery of the enzymes and their functions. In fact, these long outgrown conceptions are no longer compatible with the observed facts regarding the cells and the organism of which they are a part. The role of the enzymes in the life processes outside the alimentary canal is usually much under-emphasized, if not usually overlooked. The essential metabolic and respiratory activities occur in the cells and not in the so called digestive and respiratory organs."

Advancing knowledge in recent years of the forces acting in the living organism, has placed within the sphere of human understanding a better comprehension of the nature and characteristics of enzymes. If an intelligible opinion is to prevail regarding the true nature of enzymes, it is incumbent on all thinking men dispassionately, but with energy and thoroughness, to weigh all of the evidence and accept that which can be coordinated with established fact. Modern science cannot be satisfied with unscientific, antiquated, or untrue notions about the nature of enzymes. And I say that it is essential, in order to arrive at the truth, to weigh not only a single portion of the evidence, but all of the available chemical, medical, and biological facts together, whereby unrelated facts frequently supplement each other.

I believe the foregoing statements help to clarify the meaning of the term, "enzyme energy", or the term "enzyme activity". Enzymes must be looked upon as dual entities. This is not merely my opinion, but is the conclusion anyone must arrive at if all of the evidence is carefully considered. The sum total of biological and chemical facts does not permit formulation of a concept of the nature of enzymes based on chemistry alone. Any such concept is subject to be in error if it cannot be confirmed generally. It can be held to severe censure if at variance with widely diversified facts. It is no more unscientific to designate enzymes as consisting of protein carriers infused with energy charges, than it is improper to speak of the metallic plates and electrical energy as two separate constituents of an electrical storage battery.

Unless carefully considered, the success which has been achieved in crystallizing the protein of enzymes is liable to create an impression that some ultimate facts, at variance with the trend of the whole evidence regarding the true nature of enzymes, have been unearthed. However, I cannot see how crystallizing the protein carrier of enzymes can be interpreted as reducing enzymes to a simpler category. Even Northrop (147), Rockefeller Institute for Medical Research, one on the chief developers of the crystallization technique, admits that purely chemical methods do not solve the problem of the formation of enzymes.

Professor Willstatter (198) of Munich, Germany, in an address before the American Chemical Society at Chicago, made some remarks which have a profound bearing on this particular phase of the subject, and which will, I believe, clarify certain misconceptions that are liable to arise from time to time. I quote Willstatter: "The significance of the protein content of enzymes has become the subject of a fruitful discussion between some American colleagues and ourselves. While our own efforts in the case of saccharase, amylase, and other enzymes aimed at the gradual and, if possible, complete liberation of enzymes from protein, these American colleagues proceeded exactly in the opposite direction. They succeeded in the isolation of proteins endowed with enzymatic activity. The isolation of urease by Sumner, of pepsin by Northrop and Kunitz in the form of crystallized proteins are brilliant discoveries and important preparative successes. But it remained doubtful whether the protein content of these enzymes really forms an indispensable constituent. Dyckerhoff and Tewes in Munich and Waldschmidt-Leitz and Kofranyi in Prague were able to replace the protein, which carried peptic activity, by vegetable protein. According to these authors, the enzyme of a pepsin solution can be completely adsorbed on certain seed globulins, while the original protein component remains completely in the mother liquor without peptic activity. Thus the crystallized protein should not be considered identical with the enzyme. It cannot even be acknowledged as its indispensable colloidal carrier."

That the protein content of enzymes is not essential has been shown by Waldschmidt-Leitz and Reichel (199) who prepared amylase which was protein free.

Studies made by Giri (200) on amylase purified by adsorption with alumina gel lead to the conclusion that the enzyme is not a protein, nor does the preparation contain any determinable amount of protein.

Within recent years, enzymes have been highly purified by adsorption upon alumina gel and other substances by Sherman, Caldwell, and Adams (201). This method was originated by the Willstatter school and is extensively used in Europe. The very essence of the method indicates the dual nature of enzymes, the enzyme activity being transferred from a protein carrier to an alumina gel carrier. By the weight of these scientific demonstrations, the fact that enzymes possess incorporeal fractions is emphasized, and I propose to show that this most important part of the *enzyme complex* has *vital* characteristics.

Chapter 12

LYMPHATIC ADSORPTION AND DISTRIBUTION OF ENZYMES

The facts enumerated in the preceding few pages have an important bearing on the manner in which enzymes can be transferred about in the living organism to suit the needs of metabolism. It is commonly stated that the pancreas manufactures several hundred mL of pancreatic fluid every day, but I think it would be more appropriate to say it merely "*assembles*" this juice. It does not manufacture the water content of the juice, but derives it from the blood stream. Similarly, it does not manufacture the sodium carbonate or other salts. Whether the pancreas can manufacture out of its own substance, the amylase, protease, lipase, and other enzymes which are daily poured into the intestine is the matter principally under inquiry.

The pancreas weighs 85 grams in an adult human; the salivary glands 75 grams. At first thought, it seems absurd that a few ounces of tissue could supply from its own substance the enormous quantities of enzymes continually furnished to the intestine, one year after another. This same observation might apply with equal force to the secretions from all glands, including the endocrine glands. I do not see how it is any more logical to assume that the pancreas makes its own enzymes than it would be to state that it makes the other ingredients of its secretion. Undoubtedly, the pancreatic cells have the power to manufacture enzymes in the same degree as other cells, but certainly not in the concentration found in pancreatic secretion. I do not think there can be any dispute about where the protein constituents of enzymes come from. It can be agreed that it would be physically impossible for the pancreas to supply from its own substance, for extended periods, the protein carrier of enzymes, since this would involve rapid loss of weight and substance of the gland.

All organs, including the pancreas, participate in a loss of weight during fasting and hibernation (202). Whether the pancreas gets its protein or protein derivatives directly from the blood or indirectly from the tissues, is immaterial to this discussion. What I wish to show is that the pancreas is a collecting, transforming, and modifying organ and that it does not manufacture any of the physical components of pancreatic juice from its own substance for any great length of time, but continually receives fresh supplies. There is no reason why this same conclusion should not apply to all secreting glands. There is now only one portion of the enzyme complex left unaccounted for - the active, vital part. A studious consideration of the preceding pages makes it clear that what is variously known as *vitality, strength,* and *vital energy* as manifested by metabolic activity in the living organism, and the activity displayed by *enzymes* in altering a substrate, are one and the same thing. The pancreas appears to have the capacity of impregnating protein carriers with these vital energy values. The pancreas may be considered to function in a manner not unlike an electrical transformer which receives the electricity and changes it to such suitable voltage as may be required.

The stand that the pancreas receives all constituents of its secretion, including the vital energy faction, from the blood and tissues, is supported by all of the evidence. The mode by which enzyme energy finds its way to secreting glands has been clearly suggested by the work of German investigators.

Willstatter and Rohdewald (203) demonstrated the presence of 8 individual amylases; and also of trypsin, erepsin, and cathepsin (204) in leukocytes.

Kleinmann and Scharr (205) isolated cathepsin (pH 4 optimum) and trypsin (pH 8 optimum), from leukocytes.

Stern (206) found catalase in leukocytes, pH optimum 7.

Iglauer (207) found polymorphonuclear leukocytes to have the largest catalase content, 3 or 4 times that of erythrocytes. Eosinophilic granules showed very marked oxidase activity. Peroxidase activity was observed in leukocytes by Konn (208).

Motai (209) extracted a very active lipase with optimum pH 7.8 to 8.4 from the tonsils of dogs. The tonsils were found to be rich in lymphocytes which contained the lipase.

In an extensive investigation of tissue proteases, Kleinmann and Rona (210) ascertained that the proteases of the lymph glands are the same as those of leukocytes and suggest that the trypsin found in tissues may be derived from the destruction of leukocytes.

In the leukocytes of horse, pig, and dog blood, Willstatter and associates (204) found ereptic action for the most part strong, because of the presence of both dipeptidase and amino-polypeptidase. They consider it remarkable as to how closely the white blood cells and the pancreatic gland agree in their enzymic, especially proteolytic systems, and bring up the question whether the pancreas actually produces all of the enzyme components, or whether a process of selection and disintegration of blood cells occurs in the gland.

Willstatter and Bamann (211) extracted erepsin and cathepsin from the gastric mucosa and theorized that they occur as leukocyte enzymes in the gastric and intestinal mucosa, an assumption which was in agreement with histological observations on the accumulation of leukocytes in these tissues.

The salivary glands of dog, horse, pig, and man contain trypsin, cathepsin, and peptidase, according to the researches of Willstatter and associates (212), who consider cathepsin peculiar to the tissues and cells of the lymphoid-lymphatic system.

Careful analysis of the evidence presented places great emphasis upon hitherto unsuspected characteristics of white blood cells and makes it necessary drastically to enlarge prevailing opinion regarding their function. I have pointed out that leukocytes contain a great assortment of enzymes - perhaps greater than any other cells or tissues. Leukocytes contain a greater variety of enzymes than has been reported for the pancreas. As Willstatter called to attention, *it appears probable that white blood cells provide transportation for enzymes from place to place within the organism.* Since leukocytes are well fortified with the weapons of metabolism, the manner in which they act in phagocytosis is easier to comprehend. Certainly, it seems more feasible to believe that the vital components of enzymes discharged by the pancreas into the duodenum are brought to the pancreas from muscles and other tissues, as well as from foods and reabsorbed intestinal secretions, than it is to believe that 85 grams of pancreatic tissue can indefinitely manufacture these active enzymic fractions from its own substance.

While a toll of enzymes must be lost every day by excretion in the feces, urine, and sweat, the laws governing natural phenomena dictate that this tribute be exacted, not only from a few ounces of pancreatic, salivary, gastric, and intestinal secreting tissue, but also and perhaps mainly from the cells comprising a hundred or more pounds of muscular and glandular tissue making up the adult organism. I cannot see how this simple concept can be refuted. *Leukocytes* stand out as the most logical means of *conveyance.* Whether they pick up food enzymes and secreted enzymes in the intestinal canal by a process of adsorption; or whether the leukocytes derive their enzymes from the tissues of the organism; or whether the leukocyte enzymes come partly from one source and partly from the other are not matters concerning this particular phase of the discussion. It must be considered very likely, according to the nature of the evidence, that the pancreas and other enzyme-secreting glands receive a large portion of their enzymes from leukocytes. Perhaps, then the objection might arise that the pancreas, for instance, cannot use enzymes from various sources because of differences in hydrogen ion concentration (differences in pH) at which enzymes function.

In Northrop's (147) experiments it was shown that changing the pH of enzyme solutions and certain chemical treatments exert profound influence on certain characteristics of enzymes. Willstatter's work (148) (also see preceding references) suggests, along with that of others, that the organism has the inherent capacity of modifying various characteristics of enzymes, such as the optimum pH for maximum activity. Considering the fact that the vital fraction of enzymes may be transferred from an animal protein to a vegetable protein, as demonstrated by Dyckerhoff and Tewes and Waldschmidt-Leitz and Kofranyi; the well known adsorbtive affinity of the vital fraction of enzymes and the change in pH characteristics by treatment on enzymes with strong HCl or pepsin (Willstatter), it can be inferred that the *modification of the optimum pH for maximum activity or even change in pH characteristics, is not an insurmountable task for the organism.*

It must be remembered in this connection that the optimum pH for maximum activity of enzymes varies within wide limits with the temperature, and that the optimum temperature for maximum activity varies with the pH. As a general rule, decrease in hydrogen ion concentration (higher pH) favors increased activity at higher temperatures (50 to 70°C), and increase in hydrogen ion concentration (lower pH) favors increased activity at lower temperatures (30 to 40°C).

Compton (149) found that when takadiastase was tested at 47°C the maximum activity was at pH 7.2, while when tested at a temperature of 35.5^{o}C, its maximum activity was displayed at pH 3.

Hamburg and Pickholz (213) tested a number of different enzymes at temperatures of 38°, 60° and 70° and over a pH range from 2.8 to 8.9, and found great variations in activity.

In experiments on the dextrinization of starch, Chrzaszcz and associates (214) found the optimum pH for maximum activity of purified malt amylase to extend from pH 4.4 to pH 5.4, within a temperature range from 20°C to 75°C.

In experiments on the destruction of malt amylase by heat, I have discovered that heating a solution of the enzyme at temperatures of 48°C, 49°C, and 50°C for 1/2 hour causes a permanent increase in activity of from 7 to 15 per cent when compared with an unheated control. This increased activity is maintained even if the heated solution is kept at 5° C for 4 hours. Heating a solution of malt amylase at 51° C for 1/2 hour results in a slight loss of activity, and the loss progressively increases as heating is further increased.

In the germination of grains, α–amylase increases many times; β–amylase comparatively little (215,216). When the grain ripens, α–amylase disappears almost completely. Papaine digestion, or H2S activation, increase the β–amylase recovery from ripened grains more than 100 per cent, but there is no significant difference in the α–amylase (217). Optimum pH for α–amylase is 5.1; for β–amylase 4.3 (218). Because α–amylase disappears during ripening and is not recovered by papaine or H2S treatment, and since recovery of β–amylase is marked, it is concluded that α–amylase with optimum pH at 5.1 is convertible into β–amylase with optimum at pH 4.3. This is the conclusion also of Tychowski and Polak (218).

I believe these various phenomena are best interpreted as signifying that under the influence of complex physiological processes within the living organism, characteristics of enzymes can be modified in many ways best suited to the immediate needs of the organism. As already mentioned, the physiologist Abderhalden has recorded in a series of papers (62-71 incl.) the remarkable response of the organism in producing enzymes highly specific to various foreign substances introduced into the blood stream. Only *specific enzymes were secreted in response to sucrose, lactose, or various proteins.* Specific enzymes were isolated in the urines of animals injected with proteins or their corresponding peptones, from the following tissues of ox, horse, and dog: kidney, liver, cerebrum, cerebellum, and peripheral nerve. The proteolytic enzymes appearing in the urine were highly specific. When serum globulin was injected, the resultant enzyme would digest only serum globulin from the same blood group. Proteins from liver, kidney, pancreas, etc. similarly produced their own enzymes. Serum albumin prepared from rabbits fed on bran or green food was injected subcutaneously into bran-fed rabbits. Albumin from bran-fed rabbits produced enzymes which attacked serum albumin from bran-fed rabbits, but not serum albumin from green-fed ones.

If it be conceded that the animal body can modify characteristics of enzymes according to the dictates of necessity, the lymphatic system assumes a new order of importance. Leukocytes infiltrate the lacteals and villi of the intestine and by virtue of ameboid movement can migrate through the walls of the intestine and by a process of adsorption or absorption, or both, pick up elements of the chyle, including food enzymes and secreted enzymes, and distribute them throughout the organism. There is no good ground for denying the possibility of leukocytes absorbing enzymes since they are commonly considered to be capable of ingesting bacteria and foreign matter with which they come in contact.

Many reports credit various enzymes with bactericidal properties. It is generally agreed that leukocytes function in defense of the organism against invading agents, and, I would say, that the *defensive power of leukocytes resides in their high and diversified enzyme content*. There are many points of correlation between enzymes and leukocytes.

It must not be forgotten that both leukocytosis and increased enzyme activity occur in infectious and febrile diseases. There is a physiological leukocytosis after meals and in pregnancy, and I have pointed out that this is accompanied by a parallel rise in the enzyme content which may be detected either in the blood or urine.

Chapter 13

BODY FLUID ENZYMES IN HEALTH AND DISEASE

A severe test of the degree of dependence of the animal body on food enzymes is to determine the degree of variation or subnormality shown in the enzymes content of the blood, urine, and digestive fluids of human populations subsisting on the ordinary mixed diet. Since the average diet of individuals living under the influence of civilization is preponderantly *heat-treated* and therefore possessed of but a fraction of its original enzyme content, estimation of the enzyme content of such individuals serves as a criterion of the degree in which food enzymes are required by the organism. Fortunately, a considerable number of such series of determinations have been published for maximum health and a normal life span. The so-called normal average for enzyme content of body fluids that has been arrived at is extremely variable. This variability can be accounted for by the fact that young adults have high values because the reserve is undepleted and reactive to the extra stimulation which I have shown is an inseparable corollary of the customary diet of heat-treated carbohydrates, proteins, and fats. In older persons, the potential *enzyme tissue reserve* is more or less *depleted*. Accordingly, the body fluids display low values because of failure of the enzyme-producing mechanisms to react to stimulation.

That the enzyme content of body fluids is extremely variable in human beings of average health is abundantly shown by the literature. It is difficult to find a report where the investigator has been able to confine the results from a series of observations upon a group of individuals within reasonably narrow limits. Compared with other physiological constants, the enzyme content of a number of body juices and fluids varies within extremely wide limits. For instance, the red and white blood count, blood sugar, hemoglobin, and other blood constituents vary only within comparatively narrow limits in persons of average health. Why, then, should the enzyme content of the saliva, urine, and other fluids, in apparently normal individuals, vary 100 per cent, 200 per cent, or even as much as 1,000 per cent in many instances? These wide variations can be accounted for only on the basis of prolonged diversity in the ingestion of enzymes in food materials by different individuals. While the animal body will not tolerate a complete withdrawal of minerals or vitamins from the diet for a considerable period without manifestation of serious disease, it can live without accessory enzymes for some time and not display evidence of serious disease, although the state of health, as shown by the researches of Reyniers (219), is impaired. The animal organism cannot manufacture minerals or vitamins, generally speaking, but it can manufacture enzymes out of its own cells. The greater the demand made upon these cells for enzymes, the sooner will their power to produce them be excessively taxed or destroyed. When a certain quantity of enzymes is contributed daily by the food, the demand on the body tissues is less intense and consequently the menace of exhaustion is less formidable.

Wohlgemuth (220) was the first to observe that the amylolytic content of human saliva varies within considerable limits - 156 to 500 units. In the Japanese, Hirata (221) found a range of 160 to 640 units, using the Wohlgemuth method of analysis. In 4 adults, aged 24 to 36, Mayer (222) found a range from 200 to 2850 units in saliva, with the viscometric method. According to Gernhardt (223), there is a wide variation in the amylase content of the fasting saliva of healthy young persons. In pathological conditions, he reported still greater variations. By measurement of the reducing sugars, Emerson and Helmar (224) found 116 to 525 units in the saliva of 5 normal human controls. A remarkable experiment on the amylase content of saliva was performed recently at the Michael Reese Hospital, Chicago, Department of Gastrointestinal Research. Meyer and his associates (225), using the sugar reduction method of Hawk and Bergeim, found a variation of almost 1,000 per cent in the salivary amylase content of young adults, and only a difference of less than 300 per cent in old adults. It appears that the smaller variations in the aged may be explained on the basis that the enzyme-secreting mechanisms of the body are less susceptible to stimulation because of depletion. The amylase content in the young group was 30 times as great as in the old group. There were 12 young subjects, average age 25 years (21 to 31 years). The old group comprised 27 subjects with an average age of 81 years (69 to 100 years).

SALIVARY AMYLASE UNITS IN THE TWO GROUPS

	Range	Average
Young Group	2.4 to 22.2	10.15
Old Group	0.19 to 0.48	0.303

The Michael Reese investigators claim old people have a deficiency of starch digestion in the mouth and stomach. Young people can easily digest 50 grams of white bread in the mouth and stomach, while only 1 per cent of it will be digested in the mouth and stomach of old people. The authors of this commendable work have shown that many popular *ideas concerning the adequacy of the digestive secretions are seriously in need of revision.*

The variations in amount of amylase in urine are equally as pronounced as those in saliva. Saigusa (226) reported the amount of amylase in the urine of 114 persons varied from 6 to 64 Wohlgemuth units.

Urine amylase of 24 healthy active persons was found, by Harrison and Lawrence (227), to be from 6.7 to 33.3 Wohlgemuth units.

The urinary amylase elimination in 235 healthy persons examined by Kreyberg (228) ranged from 4 to 64 iodine units. In normal children, Morabito (229) found values of 12 to 26 for urinary amylase determined by a modification of Wohlgemuth method. Using Wohlgemuth method, Gerner (230) ascertained the amylase content in the urine of 49 healthy persons, making 114 tests. The values ranged from 16 to 128 units

Gray and Somogyi (231), using a sugar reduction method, found that in the healthy human, urine contains from 2 to 6 times as much amylase as blood serum, and that variations in amylase content are greater in urine than in blood.

In 20 normal human subjects, Dehlhougne (232) determined the enzyme concentration of blood serum. Catalase was fairly constant in normal conditions, but became extremely variable under pathological conditions. Protease showed very great variations under physiologic conditions. Peroxidase had a range of 100 per cent in normal blood and many times higher in sick persons. Esterase also had about 100 per cent variation in normals and many times greater in pathology.

Tomioka (233) gives 2.9 to 4.15 as the normal values for plasma amylase.

Elman, Arneson, and Graham (234), using the viscometer on 25 normal bloods, found 4.3 to 6.8 units for amylase.

In 5 noi mal subjects the blood amylase varied from 4.2 units to 7.2 units, using the viscometer pipette, according to Wakefield and McCaughan (235).

Morabito's (229) normal for blood amylase in children was 5 to 10 units. Harrison and Lawrence reported 3 to 7 units for the normal blood amylase in 24 healthy adults. In 49 healthy persons, 90 tests of the blood showed amylase values between 8.8 and 22.8 (reported by Gerner 230).

Reid and Myers (140), using a sugar reduction method, found the range of blood amylase content in normal individuals to be from 13 to 19 units.

Using the Ottenstein sugar reduction method, Voit and Pragal(236) gave 120 to 200 mg per 100 mL as the normal range of blood amylase content.

The concentration and total output of pepsin was studied in 21 essentially normal patients by Polland and Bloomfield (237). The maximum 10-minute volume of stomach juice digested from 16,900 to 112,400 mg of edestin.

It can be seen by the figures of those investigators reporting on both urine and blood, that the urine values vary within far wider limits than is the case with the blood. It is to be presumed that it is an inherent property of the blood stream to maintain a certain optimum concentration of enzymes, fixed within comparatively narrow limits, and that a surplus would be rapidly disposed of by deposition in the tissues or elimination in the urine. Careful blood analysis for enzymes, when properly interpreted, has diagnostic value in disease. But blood enzyme analysis in physiological research has led to the formulation of a confusing and erroneous philosophy. Examination of the digestive secretions, urine, and tissues offers the proper means of approach in tracing the course and fate of enzymes in the organism.

Many investigators have attempted to use the enzyme content of body fluids as an index to aid in diagnosis, but upon investigating a series of apparently healthy individuals in an attempt to establish a normal value, it was found that the normal range was so widely distributed that the method lost much of its diagnostic value. Two sets of factors are responsible for the wide range. Younger individuals with virgin tissues can have very high values in response to the ordinary stimulation incidental to every day living. Low values are found in old individuals with exhausted tissues. In this connection, I will seek to show that there are *many points of similarity in the chemical composition of the tissues of a comparatively young organism afflicted with degenerative disease and a comparatively old organism not so afflicted.*

It has been said that enough facts have already been unearthed by scientific research to solve many perplexing medical problems, if only these facts were properly digested and mutually related, instead of being permitted to remain buried in the vast archives of experimental literature. In the application of this doctrine to the many and varied facts on the bearing of enzymes to human health, disease, and life, I have the precept of no less a personage than Charles Darwin. If Darwin could use the method of analyzing and correlating facts to formulate a principle so fundamental and far reaching as the theory of evolution, I see no reason why this method cannot be profitably employed in establishing a concept of life, health, and disease which probably could be arrived at in no other way.

The great variation in the enzymes content of body fluids raises the question as to whether there is any relationship between the enzyme content of body tissues and fluids and chronic degenerative diseases common to middle life. While there was a wide variation in the amylase content in the fasting saliva of apparently healthy young persons examined by Gernhardt (223), in pathological conditions, he found the variation still greater. Dehlhougne (232) found 100 per cent variations in the blood content of catalase, peroxidase, and esterase of apparently healthy individuals, while, in pathology, the variations in blood content of these enzymes were many times greater. Generally speaking, many acute diseases are associated with high enzyme content of body fluids while many chronic diseases display a low content. A careful appraisal of pertinent facts supports this generalization. The incidence of low values in chronic diseases has been abundantly confirmed. Koebner (132) demonstrated a salivary lipase in several species, including man, and found it low in 7 cases of diabetes.

In gastric hypoacidity, Dehlhougne (238) found the starch splitting power of saliva much decreased.

Bettolo (239) discovered that in diabetes there is an abnormally low amylase content in the saliva.

Lipase content of serum was decreased in the cadavers of Cachectic individuals and those dying from chronic tuberculosis, according to the investigations of Bach and Lustig (117).

Ryu (240) determined that the amount of blood lipase in mild and moderate tubercular patients was about the same as normal, but in severe cases was greatly reduced, and that the reduction could be prevented if the nutritional condition was kept satisfactory.

The average blood esterase content of 111 tubercular Japanese patients was found by Sugiyama (241) to be 82 per cent lower than that of healthy individuals; and with increasing severity of the disease, the esterase activity decreased still further.

In an investigation by Balo and Lovas (242) on the enzyme content of the pancreas in 70 cadavers, *it was found that amylase, lipase, and trypsin were markedly diminished in those individuals dying of diabetes, tuberculosis, and cancer.*

Green (243) observed that when the general health was good, serum esterase content was slightly higher than normal in human cancer, but in terminal stages it was well below normal.

Determinations on the feces, blood, urine, and duodenal juice have convinced Lombardo and Anselmo (244) that protease, amylase, and lipase content is subnormal in chronic pulmonary tuberculosis. The greatest deficiency was usually of lipase.

In an unselected group of 21 cases of diabetes, Okada and associates (245) made 33 estimations on the enzyme content of the duodenal juice. There were considerable decreases in amylase, protease, and lipase in about half of the individuals.

In 5 out of 6 patients suffering from diabetes, the lipase and trypsin of the pancreatic juice were decreased according to Van Steenis (246). Analysis of feces showed incomplete digestion of meat and fats in many cases.

In a series of cases of diabetes mellitus, Sanguigno (247), Institute of Pathologic Medicine, University of Naples, found the amylase content in urine and feces to average 20 per cent below the normal, while the blood serum amylase was only 5 per cent lower.

Volodin (248), using the duodenal secretion to estimate trypsin and amylase, and blood serum and urine to test for lipase and amylase, came to the conclusion that the enzymes are usually decreased in diabetes mellitus.

The reports in the literature on the amylase content of the blood and urine in diabetes are not always consistent. After a careful study, I believe the inconsistency can be explained by consideration of the following factors:

1- *Mild cases of diabetes as a rule have high amylase values; advanced cases have low values.*
2- *Insulin exerts profound influence: it increases the amylase content of blood when low (247), and decreases it when high (140).*

3- *Carefully controlled diet of treated cases, contrasted with the unrestricted diet of untreated cases, undoubtedly exerts great influence.*

Barbera and Adinolfi (249) examined the blood, urine, and duodenal secretions in 21 cases of mild and severe diabetes. In all cases of grave diabetes the amylase content of the blood and urine was diminished.

In 29 cases of diabetes mellitus, many of them severe and untreated, Harrison and Lawrence (250) report 14 cases with a markedly lowered blood amylase content, while 15 cases had a blood amylase value low or at the lowest limit of the normal range.

Cameron (251) noted the urinary amylase content tended to be normal or subnormal in diabetes mellitus.

Paganelli (252), Institute of Medical Pathology, Camerino, reported that the amylase content of the feces was very slight in severe diabetes and almost unchanged in mild cases of diabetes.

Bassler (253) tested the duodenal contents in more than 3,000 individuals and found it possible to isolate surgical from medical gall-bladder disease and to determine the suitability of insulin in diabetes. In diabetes he found over 86 per cent of the cases were deficient in the amylase content of duodenal juice. Schmerel (254) claimed diabetic urine has a low amylase content.

Urinary amylase content was found to be reduced in diabetes by Fearon (255).

Wynhausen (256) detected considerable decrease in the amylase content in the urine of 40 diabetic individuals.

According to Brinck and Gulzow (257), the blood amylase content in diabetes mellitus is reduced.

Lewis and Mason (258) found that a severe case of diabetes may have a very low blood amylase content.

There are a number of reports relating increased amylase activity of the blood and urine in diabetes, and there is evidence that the diabetic organism may sanction an elevated blood amylase content during the earlier compensatory period of the disease. The fact that the blood amylase content is susceptible to regulation by the internal secretions has been proved. Reid and Myers (140), Reid and Narayana (259), and Cohen (260) have shown that insulin lowers the blood amylase content in man and in normal rabbits and dogs. In depancreatized dogs, Reid, Quigley, and Myers (261), and Markowitz and Hough (262) have demonstrated that insulin increases blood amylase content to the preoperative level or above it.

About half of the cases of skin afflictions, including psoriasis, *dermatitis intertriginosa*, and pruritus, examined by Ottenstein (263) showed low blood amylase values. The lowest values were found in diabetes.

In cholecystitis and diabetes, Gray and Somogyi (264) observed low values for amylase content.

Eckhardt (116) found that the urine amylase content distinctly diminished in diabetes, gastric atony, gastric anacidity, vegetative neurosis, and dystrophy.

The amylase content of the blood and urine was usually lowered in babies afflicted with nutritional disturbances (food intoxication, dystrophy, and chronic indigestion), examined by Morabito (129).

Pernice (265) observed a low blood amylase level in nutritional disorders in infants, the extent of decrease being proportionate to the severity of the disorder. He believes the blood amylase level is a useful measure of the degree of severity of diseases in infancy. It was low in dystrophies and very low in acute dyspepsia and toxicosis.

Rachmilewitz (266) examined 40 patients suffering from liver diseases for the concentration of amylase in blood serum. Of these patients 32 had jaundice. Among the conditions were catarrhal jaundice, cholangitis with jaundice, liver cirrhosis, post-dysenteric hepatitis, acute cholecystitis, and chronic cholecystitis. The blood amylase content was found to be definitely lower in liver and gall-bladder disease, particularly of long duration. He considers it of particular importance that *improvement* in the general condition of the patient, as well as of the liver function, is accompanied by a *rise* in the *amylase level* of the blood. On the other hand, progressively *deteriorating symptoms of the liver disease lead to further lowering of the amylase level.*

Kuznetzov and Michailova (267) stated that some forms of cholecystitis and cholelithiasis are not associated with decreased activity of the duodenal juice. Severe cases are. In *hepatitis parenchymatosa,* there is a lowering in efficiency of the duodenal juice. This decrease is of utmost concern in atrophic cirrhosis. In pancreatic cancer, there is a marked decrease in the quantity of duodenal juice, accompanied by a lowering of its digestive action. These investigators found that most cases of diabetes show similar conditions, as do also colitis and gastric disorders.

Hypofunction of the duodenal secretion, as evidenced by low amylolytic and tryptic activities, was encountered by Berger and associates (268) in cases of pancreatic necrosis, cholelithiasis, and cholecystitis.

In human feces, Garry (269) reported considerable diminution of amylase content in liver and gall-bladder disease, duodenal ulcer, and cancer. Polland and Bloomfield (181) believed that very low pepsin output is a more delicate index of gastric damage than low acid values.

The blood amylase content in gastric ulcer and gall-bladder disease is considerably lowered according to the figures reported by Wakefield and McCaughan (235).

In complete achylia, with negative reaction to histamine and neutral red, rennin and pepsin have been found by Schemensky and Geling (270) to be usually decreased or absent.

Probstein, Gray, and Wheeler (271) reported 9 cases of acute perforating ulcer, all of which came to operation or postmortem examination. In 4 of the cases, the ulcer involved the pancreas and in these the blood amylase content was elevated. Of the 5 cases in which the ulcer was not near the pancreas, 2 showed within the normal range, while 3 were definitely subnormal.

Several investigators claim to have found increased blood amylase content in gall-bladder disease and duodenal ulcer, and increased secretion of pepsin in duodenal ulcer. It is not inconceivable that the primary stages in these diseases may be accompanied by elevated enzyme values. There is a special reason why the enzyme content of blood and gastric juice is often found high in ulcer and gall-bladder disease. It is a universal practice to medicate digestive symptoms with alkalis. It is well known that use of alkalis in digestive disorders may lead to hypersecretion. The presence of alkali in the stomach stimulates secretion of HCl (hydrochloric acid) and pepsin. Smithies, University of Illinois College of Medicine, vigorously *condemned promiscuous use of alkalis.* Many competent physicians warn against their unsupervised use because of the danger of developing a vicious cycle of events. It is both conceivable and probable that during the initial stages of digestive disorders, use of alkalis increases the enzyme content of the stomach and blood, but when the period of exhaustion is reached, the enzyme level sinks to low values. It is a fact, for which I can supply much confirmation, that many of these salts have been proved to be excellent stimulants for secretion of enzymes. Consequently, the elevated values for enzymes sometimes reported in gall-bladder, liver, and stomach diseases are probably *induced*, rather than spontaneous.

Koehler (272) tabulated the results secured in testing the duodenal contents in 305 cases suffering from indigestion. Amylase was deficient in 26 per cent of the cases; lipase in 13 per cent; and protease in 17 per cent. In many of the cases, the oral starch tolerance or sugar tolerance test resulted in a flat blood sugar curve, in spite of the fact that the values for the 3 enzymes were normal. There is much likelihood that some of the enzymes of the small intestine, including sucrase and maltase, might be deficient, in which event it would be easy to explain the defect in carbohydrate metabolism resulting in a flat blood sugar curve after carbohydrate ingestion. Unfortunately, there are no recorded observations on the enzyme content of the secretion of the small intestine in a series of cases.

After evaluating the above evidence, there can be *no doubt that the enzyme content of the organism is daily being subjected to tremendous stress which very frequently assumes such proportions as to enhance the development of pathological phenomena.* It is only in very recent years that a few investigators have seriously considered the possibility of enzyme deficiency in the organism, and conducted tests with a view to throwing light upon an unilluminated domain. Prior to that, enzyme tests were made mainly to diagnose obstruction and malignancy of the pancreas and to determine the possibility of an excessive concentration of amylase in the serum creating excessive glycogenolysis and, perhaps, diabetes.

However, it soon became evident that diabetes could not be explained on the basis of increased amylolytic activity of the serum since in the worst cases it was very deficient, and since administration of amylase was followed by decrease in the amount of sugar excreted in the urine. The earlier investigators toyed with the idea that excessive enzyme activity in the body might account for some diseases, and conducted their investigations under this tenet. Frustration of the early attempts helped promote a better insight into the true role of enzymes in nature which crystallized in the formulation of certain fundamental concepts, with the result that investigators are now testing the *relationship of enzymes to disease with no preconceived notions.*

Chapter 14

SUBORDINATE ROLE OF ENZYMES
IN HEALTH AND DISEASE

Most investigators try to account for the observed decrease in enzyme content of blood and other body fluids by assuming that there is a failure of pancreatic function; that the pancreas becomes exhausted and is unable to continue keeping up the normal enzyme level. Professor Ivy (273), summarizing important work done at Northwestern University, said: "I suspect that a deficiency of external pancreatic secretion occurs more frequently in man than is now believed". I am sure, however, that a detailed study of the facts presented will be ample to establish conclusively that *enzyme deficiency* is not to be considered fundamentally as a depletion of the pancreas or any other enzyme-secreting organ, but as a condition originating in the tissues and *ultimately related to a decreased consumption of food enzymes occasioned by long-continued use of a heat-treated diet.* That the pancreas is only a subordinate organ in supplying enzymes is made evident when it is realized that the fall in blood enzymes consequent to experimental pancreatectomy may be made to give way to a sudden rise to the preoperative level or even above it, after injection of insulin. Such animals may live in a fair state of health for years if suitable measures are employed. From whence come these enzymes? It must be granted that under influence of endocrine guidance, the enzymes of the body are normally mobilized to be made use of according to current exigencies.

Although modern investigators, including Ivy, Oelgoetz, and Boldyreff ascribe subnormal enzyme content of the blood and digestive fluids to a failure of the pancreas per se, I believe, the literature supports the contention that the *pancreas plays only an intermediate and subordinate role and that the underlying failure and exhaustion is traceable back to the tissues* of the organism. Within recent years, it has been made plain that the organism can easily forfeit the pancreas, and if sustained by insulin and appropriate feeding, the enzyme level of the blood quickly returns to normal. This observation, confirmed by a number of researchers, has convinced them that other organs and tissues in a virgin organism can compensate for much of the work otherwise performed by the pancreas.

Wohlgemuth (33) stated that the amylase of the blood originates not only from the pancreas, but also from the intestine, salivary glands, liver, muscles, and kidneys.

Markowitz and Hough (274), Physiological Laboratory, University of Toronto, depancreatized 16 dogs and showed there was invariably a great decrease in blood amylase. But three depancreatized dogs kept alive for many months by insulin showed blood amylase values which were practically *normal*.

Using 6 depancreatized dogs, Reid, Quigley, and Myers (261) confirmed the finding of Markowitz and Hough. Following pancreatectomy there is a drop in blood amylase during the first few days and, if the animals are kept alive with insulin, it rises and may exceed the preoperative level. Withdrawal of insulin treatment invariably causes the amylolytic activity of the blood to decrease markedly.

Milla (275) ligated the pancreatic duct of dogs and found an increase of 10 to 20 times in the amylase content of blood serum and urine within 24 to 36 hours. After 10 to 15 days the amylase content returned to normal.

Ligature of the pancreatic duct in rabbits caused increase in serum amylase content and a return to normal as the gland atrophies. Gayda (276) believed not all blood amylase originates from the pancreas.

In 6 dogs, ligation of pancreatic duct by Johnson and Wies (277), Dept. of Surgery and Pathology, Yale University School of Medicine, caused a rapid increase in blood amylase content amounting to about 20 times, followed by a gradual decrease during 12 days. According to Zuckor and associates (278), in animals with ligated pancreatic ducts there is a progressive rise in serum amylase for 2 to 3 days, followed by a steep fall to nearly normal values within the next few days, after which it slowly sinks to values about half the normal.

Fiessinger and associates (279,280) could observe no significant changes in the lipase content of blood serum during 15 days following pancreatectomy in dogs.

According to Tsudzimura (281), neither pancreatectomy in the rabbit or cat, nor injection of insulin in the rabbit, affected the lipase content of the blood unless convulsions were elicited, when the lipase value rose in response to insulin.

On the other hand, ligation of pancreatic duct causes an increase in the lipase and esterase content, along with an increase in amylase. (Diena, 282)

There is no basis, therefore, for ascribing subnormal enzyme content of body fluids to failure of the pancreas, since it is seen that the virgin tissues of an organism can reestablish a normal level, and the evidence indicates that such compensation is continually at work in the virgin human organism. Because loss of the whole pancreas in an animal does not lower the serum lipase level and does not prevent the serum amylase level from returning to normal, it would be both unscientific and unwarranted to impute that failure of the human pancreas can account for frequently observed deficiencies in the enzyme content of body fluids, since, even in the worst cases, the human pancreas still contains a relatively great quantity of functioning tissue.

Pathological studies have failed to reveal disease processes in the pancreas commensurate with the magnitude of the symptoms. *Since the tissues of an experimental animal can maintain a normal serum enzyme level with the pancreas completely removed, why is not the serum enzyme level of human beings sustained with the pancreas intact?*

Chapter 15

COMPARATIVE MORTALITY OF BILIARY AND PANCREATIC FISTULAE

Professor Pearl, (283,284), Johns Hopkins University, summarized his laborious and important experiments on the duration of life in these words: "In general, duration of life varies inversely as the rate of energy expenditure during its continuance. In short, *the length of life depends inversely on the rate of living.*"

In appraising the degree of dependence of animal life upon enzymes, a convenient observation is to note the effect on health and life when enzymes are continually wasted by means of a suitably arranged fistula during the course of an experiment. A pancreatic fistula, conveying the secretion completely out of the body, offers the best means to test the ability of the organism to sustain large and continuous loss of enzymes.

If health did not suffer after a period of complete withdrawal of pancreatic enzymes from the body, it could be interpreted as signifying that enzymes are not of cardinal importance in supporting life. But if health were to show progressive decline, resulting in death, the only conclusion permissible is that the experiment demonstrates the *inviolable relation of enzymes to life* itself.

Studies on the complete drainage of pancreatic juice out of the organism have been conducted on dogs by means of pancreatic fistulae. A rapid and progressive emaciation ensued and death invariably resulted in a week or two. When special attention was devoted to maintaining the alkali reserve, life was lengthened to approximately one month. Death is usually ascribed to loss of bases. If this were the true explanation, why is it that biliary fistula is not equally fatal? A loss of fluids and salts occurs also in biliary fistula. As far as I have been able to learn, it is a general opinion among surgeons of experience that the prognosis in human pancreatic fistula is far more speculative than is that in human biliary fistula. The main difference between pancreatic fistula and biliary fistula, regarding their influence on life, as I see it, is that in pancreatic fistula there is a steady *sacrifice of enzymes*, whereas no such loss occurs in biliary fistula.

Colp (285) analyzed 61 cases of human external duodenal fistulae and found the mortality averaged 51 per cent. He thinks the loss of fluids alone cannot account for the rapid debilitation which occurs with loss of the enzyme-containing secretions, for even though the body is supplied sufficiently with fluids, deterioration occurs.

Berg and Zucker (286) excluded the pancreatic juice from the intestine of dogs by means of external fistulae and reported death took place in 7 to 56 days. After varying periods of loss of pancreatic juice, the dogs lost their appetite, declined rapidly in weight, showed marked weakness and apathy, developed a bloody diarrhea, and finally succumbed.

Laqua (287) found that while continued deprivation of the duodenal juice and bile does not endanger life in dogs, complete loss of pancreatic secretion regularly leads to an early death.

Total drainage of pancreatic juice from the body results in death of dogs within 5 to 8 days, according to the experiments of McCaughan (288). Dehydration, weakness, anorexia, and vomiting preceded death. Postmortem examination was invariably negative. The use of the whole juice by mouth produced a spectacular change and apparently restored a moribund dog to a normal state within a few hours.

In 7 dogs with Thiry fistulae, the continued loss of *succus entericus* in response to intestinal distention caused a change in its chemical composition, in experiments undertaken by Herrin (289), Dept. of Physiology, University of Wisconsin. There was a decrease in chlorine and fixed base and a great increase in bicarbonate. The serum showed a decrease of 26 per cent in chlorine, 20 per cent in bicarbonate, and 10 per cent in fixed base. Anorexia, followed by circulatory failure, coma, and death developed in about 4 days.

Walters, Kilgore, and Bollman (290) found that if a sufficient volume of water is added to NaCl (common salt) and the solution given twice daily in experimental fistula, life may be maintained 3 weeks or longer. During this time the blood chlorides are raised to their normal level, and the accumulation of non-protein Nitrogen in the blood is prevented.

In Bottin's (291) experiments on dogs, the complete loss of pancreatic secretion caused death within 21 to 40 days, rather than within 8 days as reported by earlier investigators using less careful technique. Progressive dehydration, demineralization, and acidosis developed.

Regarding biliary fistulae, Hawkins and Whipple (292) reported that it is possible, with care, to keep a bile fistula dog in a normal state for months or years if proper attention is given to the diet and physical state. Dogs with renal type biliary fistulae have been under observation in the laboratory of Hawkins and Whipple in perfect health for many years.

The survival period of 12 dogs, operated on to produce complete biliary fistulae by Thanhauser and associates (293), Tufts Medical College, averaged 6 weeks, with no special diet or care.

Heymann (294) arranged biliary fistulae in 3 puppies, 6 to 7 weeks of age. The animals continued to gain weight, though at a slower rate for 4 to 6 weeks after the operation, followed by a progressive loss in weight that finally led to cachexia and death. No particular attention was given to diet or care.

Howell (42) states that it is an interesting physiological fact that some patients in whom the entire supply of bile has been diverted to the exterior, may still continue to enjoy fair health.

It must be pointed out that, even with the best of care, continuous loss of pancreatic juice is rapidly fatal, while with the same kind of care complete loss of bile is tolerable and compatible with fair health. There is no alternative but to ascribe the dire consequences of a loss of pancreatic juice to the sacrifice of enzymes which are *necessary* in many ways to the normal functioning of organisms.

Chapter 16

RELATION OF ENZYME POTENTIAL TO RESISTANCE AND LONGEVITY

Throughout the past, there has been no physical means of identifying and measuring vital forces. Science could recognize that there was such an entity as vitality, but it was not possible to form more than a vague image of its nature. It is no longer warranted to consider vitality and life energy as intangible forces. The available evidence does not justify a placid continuance of a nihilistic attitude toward the vital forces operating in the living organism. It is a motif of science to reduce complex phenomena to simple integral units. Enzymes emerge as the true yardstick of vitality. Enzymes offer the only means of calculating the vital energy of an organism. That which has been referred to as "vitality", "vital force", "vital energy", "vital activity", "nerve energy", "nerve force", "strength", "vital resistance", "life energy", "life", and "life force", may be and probably is synonymous with that which has been known as "enzyme activity", "enzyme value", "enzyme energy", "enzyme vitality", and "enzyme content." The available evidence does not permit further procrastination but requires that what is known, vaguely and incomprehensibly, as *life force or activity be defined in terms of concrete and measurable enzyme units.* In the face of the evidence which I present, it would be unscientific to continue fostering an unintelligible and uncertain attitude on matters having wide and intense bearing upon human conduct.

The data which I am about to present will demonstrate the true nature of what we know as life energy and vitality, and reduce these ethereal entities to dimensional proportions. A scientist is not only a man who must observe and measure facts, but, if his work is to have constructive value, it is incumbent on him also to coordinate facts. Otherwise, they may stand useless and barren as a mountain of rock.

Evidence bearing on the influence of various factors controlling the output of vitality in an organism upon the length of life arranges itself into several groups:

1. *Effect of temperature on the speed of metabolism and length of life*: In pecilothermic organism, higher temperatures make for more rapid metabolism and a shorter life span.
2. *Effect of degree of activity on length of life*: Increasing the heart rate decreases length of life.
3. *Effect of quantity of food intake on length of life*.

It is a matter of common observation among biologists that cold-blooded organisms, when exposed to high temperatures, become very active and soon succumb. At low temperatures they are sluggish, but live much longer. It is known that the activity of enzymes likewise increases with elevation of the temperature, and the evidence indicates that at an elevated temperature the enzyme content of an organism is more rapidly spent, and therefore life must end sooner. *The increased metabolic activity with rise in temperature can be explained only on the basis of increased enzyme activity. Increased rate of enzyme depletion begets a shorter life span.* In the event of freedom from disease and a sufficient food supply, death can be ascribed solely to enzyme depletion; and there is evidence that the exhaustion need not be total.

Pepper (295), Montana Agric. Exper. Station, held adults of the confused flour beetle, *Tribolium confusum*, at a temperature of 118 degrees F for 10 hours and made 10 catalase determinations at hourly intervals. The results showed a gradual inactivation of the enzymes, but no abrupt change took place in this general trend even after 100 per cent mortality had been produced. Pepper noted that when insects are exposed to high temperatures they become very active at first and then gradually become dormant and appear to be dead.

I have found *118 degrees F to be a critical temperature.* The human skin can withstand a temperature of 117 degrees F for many hours; 118 degrees F gradually produces uncomfortable stimuli, while 119 degrees F causes a superficial burn. It has also been found that seeds will not germinate if the enzyme content has become diminished beyond a certain point.

Marquis wheat seeds were heated at various temperatures for one half hour in a thermostatically controlled bath, after being soaked in water for 12 hours. There were 50 seeds in each group. After heating, the seeds were allowed to germinate between wet blotter paper. I have made a number of such experiments, using different seeds. Always the results have been similar. The number of seeds germinated, out of 50, were:

Temperature °F	Number Germinated
Unheated	43
118	34
122	25
126	15
129	none
133	none

The influence of mild increase in temperature in promoting increased metabolism and shortened duration of life is shown in an interesting way when insects are maintained at different temperatures and their life spans determined. Loeb and Northrop (296), Rockefeller Institute for Medical Research, maintained aseptic fruit flies (Drosophila) at various temperatures. The following table gives the duration of life in days:

Temperature °C	Larval Stage Days	Pupal Stage Days	Imago Days	Total duration of life from egg To death in days
10	57.0	-	120.5	177.5
15	17.8	13.7	92.4	123.9
20	7.77	6.33	40.2	54.3
25	5.83	4.23	28.5	38.5
30	4.12	3.43	13.6	21.15

Water fleas, *Moina Macrocopa Strauss*, were kept separately in vials containing 25 mL of culture medium at various temperatures, and the duration of life reported by Terao and Tanaka (297) is as follows:

Temperature °C	Duration of life Days
15	14.36
21	9.28
27	6.5
33	4.7

MacArthur and Baillie (298), Dept. Biology, University of Toronto, determined the influence of temperature on longevity in *Daphnia Magna* and gave the following results:

Temperature °C	Duration of life Days
8	108.2
10	87.8
18	40.0
28	25.6

The male life span extended from 21.9 days at 28 degrees to 107.9 days at 8 degrees, an increase of 492 per cent. The female life span lengthened from 29.2 days to 108.4 days, an increase of 373 per cent. *Longevity varied as an inverse function of temperature between 8 and 28 degrees C.* The temperature coefficient had a value of 2.12, which the authors stated closely approximates that for most chemical reactions. They concluded that the effects of sex and temperature upon longevity were such as would be expected if average duration of life, in the absence of genetic differences, was regulated chiefly by metabolic rates.

Careful measurements of the energy metabolism with the calorimeter during incubation of hens' eggs have been made by Barett (299), United States Dept. of Agriculture. Under controlled conditions of temperature, humidity, carbon dioxide, and oxygen content, the duration of time required for hatching at different temperatures was:

Temperature °F	Time required To hatch
96	23 days, 13 hours
98	21 days, 13 hours
99	20 days, 20 hours
100	20 days, 5 hours
102	19 days, 11 hours
103.5	19 days, 4 hours

The appearance of the chicks varied with the temperature. At 102 degrees, they were not so large, fluffy, or lively as at 99 or 100 degrees. Many abnormalities, such as crooked necks and sprawling legs, appeared in chicks hatched at the higher temperatures. Measurement of heat elimination, carbon dioxide elimination, and oxygen consumption showed conclusively, according to Barett's extensive tabulations, that the metabolic activity is at a considerably higher tempo at the higher temperatures. The higher temperatures engendered a higher energy metabolism, and consequently development and emergence of the chicks was more rapid.

In experiments conducted on cantaloupe seedlings, Pearl (300), Institute for Biological Research, Johns Hopkins University, showed that seedlings which have a relatively rapid rate of CO_2 production in respiration during the growing period, and which metabolize a relatively large amount of dry matter and of water during growth, live a shorter time in total than do seedlings which have a relatively small metabolic transfer of dry matter and water during growth. The relatively long-lived plants lived at a slower rate than the relatively short-lived plants.

Gowen (301) found CO_2 production in 4 groups of *Drosophila melanogaster* inversely proportional to length of life.

Bodine (302), Zoological Laboratory, University of Pennsylvania, determined the curves for CO_2 output and catalase content in grasshoppers, *Chortophaga viridifasciata*, potato beetles, *Leptinotarsa decemlineata*, and fireflies were approximately parallel, indicating variation in the same direction. The catalase content decreased with increasing age.

In both sexes of *Daphnia Magna*, MacArthur and Baillie (303) observed that a change in temperature from 8 to 28 degrees increased the heart rate 412 per cent, increased direct susceptibility to KCN (Potassium Cyanide) 435 per cent, and shortened the life span 423 per cent. *In both sexes, the life span was condensed or lengthened as the average metabolic level was raised or lowered.* The average heart rate per second was:

Temperature °C	Heart rate Per second
8	1.69
18	4.26
28	6.84

Quoting above authors: "The observed duration of life of males was shorter than that of females by an amount equal to that by which their observed metabolic rates exceeded those of the females. Nearly the same total number of heart beats, some 15,400,000 occurs in a daphnid's life, regardless of temperature or sex. The organism appears to receive a specific sum total of 'vitality,' rather than a definite allotment of days. It is the tempo of life or rate of energy expenditure which determines aging of organisms. Duration of life varies inversely with the intensity of the metabolism. *Life runs out its course* to its natural term with a velocity directly proportional to the catabolic rate or, as commonly expressed, according to rapidity of *'wear and tear'*".

In an address before the New York Academy of Medicine, Professor Pearl compared certain characteristics of two groups of white men, 193 in each group, observed until all had died. *One group lived an average of 26 years longer* per individual than the other. Certain important differences of the long-lived group were:

1. *Pulse rate 4 beats less per minute.*
2. *Weight 6 pounds each lower.*
3. *Smaller chest girth at expiration.*
4. *Smaller waist at the navel level.*

It is not true, Pearl said, that the absolute length of life has lengthened. Actually fewer persons of 70 today survive to an age of 90 compared to 40 years ago. The lengthened life span of today is due to saving the lives of more babies and children.

Albergo (304) studied the basal metabolic rates in 22 subjects aged 59 to 85 years, all in good general health, and found, in most cases, a lowered B.M.R. as compared with the average in 5 normal controls, aged 22 to 40. The rise in metabolism after food was likewise less in old age than in middle age.

McCay (305) believes, as a result of long-term rat experiments, that longevity and maximum growth are incompatible.

McLester (306) pointed out that most physiologists would consider the increased rate of growth in relation to so-called improved nutrition as wholly favorable. Increased stature of Chinese and Japanese living in California is ascribed to more abundant food. A study made recently at four womens' colleges - Vassar, Wellesley, Smith, and Mount Holyoke - showed that daughters of former students were about 1 1/8 inches taller than their mothers. The 1935 graduating class at Barnard averaged 1/2 inch taller than the class of 1925. It has also been stated that the recorded weights of Wistar Institute albino rats are higher than some 20 years ago (307). It is alleged that this is brought about by improved and more abundant food supply.

There appears to be no scientific substantiation for the popular belief that rotundity in infants and increased weight and stature in adults are evidence of optimum health. The evidence, actually, points to the opposite conclusion. Northrop (308), Rockefeller Institute for Medical Research, prolonged the larval period in the aseptic fruit fly (Drosophila) by inadequate feeding and observed an increase in the total duration of life from 19.3 days to 28.9 days. The larval stage increased from 8 days to 17 days.

Using a synthetic diet (essentially enzyme free), properly supplemented, McCay and associates (1), Animal Nutrition Laboratory, Cornell University, divided 106 white rats into three groups:

Group No. 1 was allowed all the feed desired.

Group No. 2 was restricted in feed intake from the time of weaning.

Group No. 3 was allowed sufficient feed to permit normal growth for 2 weeks after weaning and then restricted in the same manner as group No. 2.

Average life span of male rats in days

Group No. 1- Unrestricted food intake	483 days
Group No. 2- Restricted food intake	820 days
Group No. 3- Partially restricted food intake	894 days

The Cornell work is part of a long-term undertaking commenced some 10 years ago and still proceeding. After reviewing this work, I cannot see how it is possible to escape the conclusion that when the *enzyme reserve* (I use this phrase interchangeably with the term vitality) *is drawn at a more rapid rate it will be exhausted sooner and consequently life will end earlier.*

Large groups of brook trout have been stunted by McCay and associates (309) for periods exceeding 20 weeks, both by feeding synthetic rations with low protein levels and by means of restricted allowances of raw meat. Trout stunted with low protein levels lived twice as long as those that were allowed to grow upon similar synthetic rations but at higher protein levels.

Ingle and his collaborators (310), Brown University and Carnegie Institution, working with *Daphnia longispina*, arrived at some important conclusions regarding the influence of quantity of food upon the life span and the speed of metabolism. The diet was not subjected to any artifices, such as heat treatment. It was shown that increase in quantity of food produced a higher rate of metabolism, as evidenced by increase in speed of the heart, and thus the individuals completed the life cycle in a shorter time. Animals were maintained individually at

25 degrees C in 100 mL of nutritional medium. Starved animals were maintained in a low nutritional level of medium consisting of one part of normal medium to 36 parts of pond water. The average life span of 158 well-fed individuals was 29.60 days; the average for 141 "starved" animals was 39.19 days - an increase of about 40 per cent. The heart beat frequency at birth averaged 4.68 beats per second. In well-fed individuals, the rate reached a maximum of 5.46 beats per second, after which it dropped gradually and at time of death was only 3.4 beats per second. In the starved animals, the heart rate at death averaged 4.38 beats per second, which was almost one beat per second more than that of well-fed animals. This showed that the vitality of the starved individuals was not yet exhausted and that they could have lived still longer with an optimum level of nutrition.

Ingle's results, in the main, corroborate Rubner's hypothesis that *length of life is dependent upon a definitely limited sum total of energy which the organism has to expend*, and life normally ends when the energy limits have been reached. It follows that, if an organism dissipates its supply of energy quickly, death occurs sooner than if the energy is expended slowly. This view of Rubner's has been confirmed in such diverse ways that no doubt should remain. However, it is no longer necessary or desirable to denote the energy of an organism as an abstract entity. Failure to recognize the identity and oneness of enzymes and vital energy impedes the development of a clearer understanding of what constitutes health, disease, and life, and is in the end injurious to an optimal state of health.

The fact that the enzyme content of organisms is depleted with increasing old age is reinforced when the fluids or tissues are examined at different ages. After full mature growth has been attained, there is a slow and gradual decrease in the enzyme content of organisms. When the enzyme content becomes so low that metabolism cannot proceed at a proper level, death overtakes the organism.

Burge and Burge (311), University of Illinois, attributed the increase in respiratory metabolism or oxidation in youth, and its decrease in old age, to the increase and decrease, respectively, of the *tissue catalase*.

They measured the catalase content of the whole bodies and eggs of Colorado potato beetles, with the following results:

Unfertilized egg	18
Fertilized egg	35
Newly hatched larva	280
Quarter grown larva	800
Half grown larva	1,250
Three-quarter grown larva	1,725
Full grown larva	1,750
Pupa	1,800
Adult Beetle	1750
Old beetle	900

Bodine (312) found that the catalase content in adult grasshoppers, *Chortophaga viridifasciata*, potato beetles, *Leptinotarsa decemlincata*, and fireflies, decreased with increasing age.

Sekla (313), Dept. of General Biology and Experimental Morphology, Charles University, Prague, determined the esterase content in *Drosophila Melanogaster* of different ages and types. Previously Pearl had found the vestigial *Drosophila Melanogaster* to have a mean duration of life of 20 days, while the mean duration of life in the wild type was 46 days. Measurements of the esterase and protease content of extracts of the whole bodies of these flies have shown that the content of these enzymes is considerably greater in the long-living type than in the short-living vestigial type. Measurements revealed the esterase content is least in flies 1 day old. In a population containing all the flies emerging in the course of 10 days the content markedly increases. After this, the extract of flies 25 days old shows a decrease in esterase content, the figures approaching those of the flies emerged.

The ester-hydrolyzing or lipase actions of extracts of whole macerated rats, whose ages ranged from 3 days before birth to 3 years 15 days, were tested on 10 simple esters by Falk, Noyes, and Sugiura (314). For the embryo and the youngest rats, the activity was minimal, increasing in adult rats. As age advanced, the enzyme content diminished, reverting to the same content as the embryonic type for the oldest rats.

Mayer (315) studied the amylase content of human saliva at different ages and arrived at the following results:

	Number of Cases	Average Amylase Value
Infants-premature	2	26
Infants-1 to 3 days old	2	50
Babies-7 to 18 months	2	370
Adults-24 to 36 years	4	1,045

Finizio (316) found the amylase content of saliva increased progressively in infants till the age of 12 months. At 8 to 10 months it had doubled. At 1 year it was a trifle less than that of children of 2 or 3 years.

Meyer and co-workers (317), Dept. of Gastrointestinal Research, Michael Reese Hospital, Chicago, found the salivary amylase in 12 individuals, 21 to 31 years of age (average age 25), to be 30 times as great as that of 27 individuals, 69 to 100 years old (average age 81).

Loeschke (318), University Pediatric Clinic, Cologne, Germany, Determined that the amylase content of blood depends on age and it is especially small in premature infants.

According to Pernice, (319), Pediatric Clinic, Marburg, Germany, the blood amylase in infants increases with age, being very low in premature infants. The increase is rapid until the age of 6 months and the lower level for adults is reached at 1 year.

The amylase content of blood and urine was found by Morabito (229) to be slight in children compared to adults.

McClure and Chancellor (320) reported the following values for amylase content of children's urine:

FIRST YEAR	0.0 TO 10.0
SECOND YEAR	2.5 TO 06.6
THREE TO SEVEN YEARS	0.8 TO 10.0
SEVEN TO FIFTEEN YEARS	5.0 TO 20.0

Eckhardt (115) (116) tested 1,200 urine specimens from human subjects of all ages for amylase content. Especially low values were found in early infancy. The mean value for all ages was about 20. In adolescents the range was 10 to 40, while in old age it was lower, from less than 8 to 20.

Dhar (321,322), Chemical Laboratory, Allahabad University, India, believes animal life depends essentially on the catalytic activity of enzymes in the animal body and compares it to the catalytic decomposition of hydrogen peroxide in the presence of manganese dioxide. This is much greater if a freshly prepared sample of manganese dioxide is used. *Old age is considered by Dhar to be due to decrease in enzyme activity and consequently lowered metabolism.*

The foregoing evidence makes it clear that age is not so much a matter of days or years, but depends altogether on the physical condition of the tissues. It is common experience among physicians to find individuals of 60 years with a physical inventory characteristic of persons of 40, and vice versa.

Ingle and associates (310) pointed out that senescence in *Daphnia longispina*, manifested by more sluggish movements, declining heart rate, irregular wrinkling of the carapace, failure of reproduction, gradual decrease in length of the caudal spine, and some decrease in body size, is attained much earlier in well-fed individuals than in those on restricted feed. Quotation: "As late as the 18th instar, starved Daphnia are potentially young animals, as is indicated by the fact that if the proper environmental conditions are afforded them at that time they exhibit growth, reproduction, heart rate, and instar duration characteristics of relatively young animals. Furthermore, to the experienced worker, they appear young and show none of the indications of senescence observed in the well-fed group." Upon reflection, it will be seen that *wrinkling of the skin, decrease in height and weight, lowered physical activity, and metabolism and similar evidence of enzyme depletion in senile human beings, closely parallel the observed phenomena in senile Daphnia* induced by a high level of metabolism and therefore the extra burden on the enzyme reserve.

Gafafer (323) reported measurements on the rate of growth of about 30,000 school children. About half the children had some physical defect such as caries, goiter, defective tonsils, adenoids, defective vision, or enlarged lymph glands, but none was seriously ill. It was found the nondefectives had shorter trunks and smaller chest girths, thus showing that there is a tendency to incompatibility between maximum physical development and optimal health. It may be recalled that Pearl had found persons with smaller chest girths to live longer than those with larger chest girths.

Simms and Stolman (324), Columbia University School of Medicine, analyzed the kidney, liver, heart, spleen, and muscle of 6 persons of 70 years or above and 11 persons between 30 and 40 years old. Increase in age was accompanied by increase in the Cl, Na, Ca, total base, and (except in the heart) H_2O contents of the tissues; and by decrease in the K, Mg, P, N, and ash contents (except in liver). Changes of the same kind were found when organs of old and young persons who had died of disease were analyzed. Comparison of the mineral composition of the tissues of healthy and diseased persons of the younger group showed that *in disease, changes similar to those occurring in old age tended to take place.*

In a study of 4,205 human individuals, it was shown by Bernstein (325) that early development of presbyopia was associated with an early termination of life. Later development of presbyopia was associated with longer life. With increasing age, there was increase in the cholesterol and insoluble globulins, associated with loss of water and hardening of the lens, thereby changing accommodation and producing presbyopia.

Chapter 17

INCIDENCE OF DISEASE IN ANIMALS

Extemporaneous opinion as to the incidence of disease in wild animals is not consistent. Some will say that wild animals develop many diseases; others that wild animals in their natural habitat are singularly free from all diseases. I have been unable to find recorded evidence of any instance of a pathological condition in wild jungle animals. When wild animals were held in captivity for exhibition purposes, it was customary, until recent years, to use a random diet, especially for the carnivora and omnivora. The diet included generous quantities of white bread, boiled potatoes, and cooked meat. Raw food was at a premium. Therefore the intake of *food enzymes* was *drastically curtailed* and the *drain upon tissue enzymes* correspondingly increased. The *high mortality* in past years of valuable zoo animals is well known to those responsible for maintenance of these animals. It was impossible to preserve life in anthropoids in captivity for more than a short time. Reproduction was not often successful and the raising of young a perilous undertaking, especially in carnivora. Conditions have now changed. Valuable animals are given mostly raw food and little or no heat-treated food. At the Lincoln Park Zoo in Chicago, famous for its low mortality, tigers and lions are fed raw meat and bones exclusively with an occasional addition of raw liver. Anthropoids are given bananas, apples, oranges, and raw vegetables. No cooked material of any nature is used. The change in the health of captive wild animals has been remarkable. Reproduction and rearing of young are now regularly successful even among the anthropoids, which are now maintained indefinitely in captivity. Deaths are few and far between among large animals. Five years ago, I tried to get dissection material for the study of organ weights in large carnivorous animals and was told that deaths among tigers and lions are now relatively infrequent, sometimes several years elapsing before a specimen becomes available. There has been no significant change in the living conditions among these animals save only the character of the food; increased use of raw, uncooked food. Any *improvement in health* standards of captive wild animals must accordingly be ascribed to something that *raw food* possesses and which is not found in heat-treated food. Enzymes claim the distinction of being the only factors present in *raw foods* and completely lacking in heat-treated food. Improvement in health and decrease in mortality among inhabitants of zoos can only be explained on the basis of larger consumption of food enzymes.

When it becomes necessary to maintain health and life in a valuable animal for the maximum duration of time, something more than ordinary heat-treated diet is necessary, even though sufficient quantities of vitamins and minerals are added to it. All zoos are now using raw diets more or less and those using most raw food have the lowest mortality.

The incidence of disease in wild animals in captivity has been carefully studied by Dr. Fox, Pathologist to the Zoological Society of Philadelphia. In his volume on the subject is to be found an extensive tabulation, accompanied by microphotographs, of more than 5,000 autopsies on animals and birds which had died during some 20 years up to the year 1923. During this period of time, modern dietary practices had not yet been inaugurated and the incidence of pathological conditions common to man was large. At least 30 common pathological entities were defined, many by tissue diagnosis. Among those found were, acute and chronic gastritis, duodenitis, enteritis, colitis, liver disease and nephritis, myocardial degeneration, pernicious anemia, thyroid disease, arthritis, malignancy, tuberculosis, arterial disease and adrenal disease.

It seems to be the opinion, at least in some quarters, that such an imposing array of pathological conditions is not to be found in modern zoos since the dawn of the raw diet principle. *It is interesting to note that when captive wild animals are fed a diet resembling human food in the sense of it being largely heat-treated, they develop diseases similar or identical to those found in human beings.*

Brown, Pearce, and Van Allen (103), Rockefeller Institute for Medical Research, studied the weights of 17 organs in several hundred rabbits with reference to the influence of minor abnormalities, lesions, and disease on organ weights. The rabbits were 8 to 12 months old, purchased from dealers and caged 2 to 8 weeks. Their past history was unknown. It was found that many rabbits displayed minor lesions of various organs. This might be cited to uphold the theory that there is a certain degree of prevalence of disease among wild animals. However, it is not possible to take this attitude when all factors are considered. The fact that the progenitors of domesticated rabbits have been extensively used in laboratory experimentation for many years and for many rabbit generations, alone condemns the rabbit as a representative of undefiled wild life. Many times adult experimental animals or the offspring of experimental animals find their way to dealers and commercial breeders. The Wistar Institute of Anatomy and Biology has recognized and met this need for animals with an unambiguous history. Not only is their genealogy open to suspicion, but the diet of rabbits while in the dealers' pens is diverse and often unsatisfactory. Table scraps, including bread and other heat-treated foods, often form a large part of the diet. In this way it is possible to account for the lesions described by the Rockefeller workers, some of which I have personally observed in rabbits.

In a study of obscure lesions in 350 normal rabbits, it was found by the Rockefeller workers (103) that so long as the animals were in apparently good health the organ weights did not differ materially from those animals that were entirely free from lesions. There were, however, slight changes which suggest functional responses similar in character to the more marked changes in mass that occur in rabbits showing clinical symptoms of disease.

In a group of 127 rabbits, manifesting disease of spontaneous origin, the same investigators (104) found decided changes in the weights of nearly all organs; changes which appeared to be of functional origin.

In a group of 295 normal rabbits, the Rockefeller investigators (105) found that disease, even in its mildest form, is capable of influencing the weights of organs that are not directly involved in the disease process, and that the effect produced bears a relation to both the extent and the activity of the lesions present.

For $2^1/2$ years, Orr and his colleagues (326), Rowett Research Institute, Aberdeen, kept half of a large rat population on a diet equivalent to that of a human population, including 25 common articles of food cooked in water. The other half received, in addition, green food and as much milk as they cared to drink. From birth to weaning, there was a total of 1,211 rats on the human diet and 1,706 on the supplemented diet. Those on the human diet showed a lower blood hemoglobin, slightly impaired reproductivity, increased susceptibility to infection, and a clinically poorer condition as measured by behavior and the state of coat. Enteritis, pneumonia, anemia, and pericarditis were frequently observed at examination and post mortem. The authors suggest that the findings indicate a *large section of the human population may be far from optimal in the nutritional content of their diet.*

In nutritional experiments on rats with a synthetic diet, supplemented by addition of vitamins (relatively enzyme free) and salts, McCay and associates (1) observed many pathological conditions such as tumors and diseases of the lungs, kidneys, and genital tract. Quotation: "In the course of nearly four years in which this experiment was in progress, many different pathological conditions were observed that are rarely seen in rat colonies. This was due to the maintenance of old animals in contrast to the usual breeding colony for rats where individuals are usually discarded shortly after middle life. The roughness of the fur coat became apparent much earlier in those that matured rapidly. As the experiment progressed many animals became blind; a rough estimate would include at least half of the animals living beyond 2 years. Old rats were frequently afflicted with diseases of the urinary tract. At times bloody urines were encountered."

Dr. V.G. Heiser in a recent talk to the National Association of Manufacturers told of experiments on 4,000 rats in which half were fed on a natural diet and the other half received the kind of food the average family uses. At the end of two years, the first group was essentially free from disease while the group partaking of human diet, was afflicted with a number of diseases including gout, gastric ulcer, arthritis, and tuberculosis.

As McCay suggests, the average experiment designed to test the vitamin value of some particular article is of short duration and offers no clue as to the sufficiency of a diet, however well it may be supplemented by vitamins. In order to prove the hypothesis that a diet perfectly balanced by minerals and the known vitamins can maintain health, it would be necessary to use synthetic, purified rations and continue the diet during the whole life span of the animal. It is not to be expected that serious ill-health or disease would ordinarily make an appearance except during the latter period of life, and furthermore, judgment as to state of health should not be limited to visual inspection or considerations of weight. From what has preceded, it can be seen that ra :e of weight increment is worthless as a criterion of the true health of an animal and of its chances for long life. Indeed, it can be pointed out that far from having a desirable influence, a weight premium is a handicap and offers a means of forecasting an early senility. In the Cornell undertaking of McCay, Crowell, and Maynard (1), it was shown that the animals attaining maximum weight first died early, while those reaching their greatest weight later lived a much longer life. Their results follow:

	Average Life Span Days	Mean Maximum Weight attained
Unrestricted food intake	483	439
Restricted food intake.	820	262
Partially restricted food intake	894	267

Jespersen and associates (327) concluded that feeding raw potatoes is uneconomical in preparing pigs for market because the pigs are too old before they reach the slaughter weight. Cooked potatoes proved more efficient.

Thompson and Hargrave (328) found the pigs receiving steamed potatoes as part of their ration grew more rapidly than those receiving raw potatoes and that the advantage amply repaid the cost of steaming the potatoes.

Chapter 18

EFFECTS OF RAW OR PASTEURIZED MILK

However valuable vitamins may be in specific instances, the attempt to balance synthetic diets with vitamins and minerals but without enzymes has already ended in failure. Increased use of vitamins has not retarded the incidence of, or rising death rates from several serious diseases, nor is there any evidence that purified vitamin preparations can produce other than temporary effects except in a few specific conditions.

The prevalent idea that raw food has no virtue except that it supplies vitamins and minerals is a serious menace to human health. Canners are exploiting this notion for commercial reasons. It is pointed out that canned food has sufficient vitamins and any slight deficiency can be easily made up by use of vitamin preparations. It has been claimed that the survival of the human race on a diet consisting of an abundant amount of cooked food offers a satisfactory rebuttal to the doctrine that raw food is necessary to maintain a satisfactory level of health. But the human being cannot be accepted as symbolic of a healthy organism. The average human life span does not measure up to biological standards. Superficial evidence of early degenerative changes in human beings is clearly discernible by anyone. The prevalence of caries, nasopharyngeal abnormalities, and postural defects among children; excessive hair loss, eye defects, and skin lesions in young adults; and various functional or serious organic diseases in later life; disqualifies man as a prototype of reasonably good health. Incessantly mounting death rates in most degenerative diseases speak against the theory that the prevalent use of large quantities of heat-prepared food by man is normal or optimal.

Certainly, there is no necessity of further prompting or urging to increase the use of cooked food in human diet. And yet, that is the very tendency among certain vitamin investigators. Recently Kohlman, Eddy, White, and Sanborn (329), Research Laboratories National Canners Association, and Teachers College Columbia University, published results of some experiments to test the comparative value of canned, home-cooked, and raw food diets. Through 5 generations, close to 500 rats were reared on each diet. The weights of animals on the canned diet were greatest. This is no particular virtue and is what might be expected of any heat-treated food, particularly carbohydrates, for reasons which have already been discussed. Otherwise, the experiment proves nothing except that rats can reproduce on a cooked diet, which fact had already been repeatedly demonstrated on animals as well as by human experience. The animals were evidently discarded after reaching 90 days of age since no further data is recorded. From the extensive evidence I have submitted, one can gather it would manifestly be a grave error to make deductions as to the efficacy of a particular type of diet in the maintenance of continued good health and freedom from disease on the basis of information elicited during the first 90 days of the life of the rat - the period of adolescence - comprising about 1/8 of the life span. And yet the above investigators try to establish the sufficiency and even virtue of cooked foods in these words: "Certainly, the idea that a certain amount of raw food is absolutely indispensable to health might well be questioned in the face of such evidence. If cooking does not alter chemical compounds to prevent their playing their particular role in nutrition, cooking from this standpoint cannot be decried. Cooking inactivates plant enzymes. Their activity in a ruptured raw plant cell is generally not wholesome; that conditions should be such in the digestive tract as to make it wholesome is scarcely to be expected". This is a direct implication that the activity of plant enzymes in the digestive tract, after foods are chewed and swallowed, becomes unwholesome and that a logical safeguard is use of cooked or canned food. The experiment was evidently a strained attempt to stimulate increased use of canned foods and all questions raised by it are fully answered in this manuscript. It is evident that these particular investigators have not reviewed the great body of evidence to be found in periodical literature. Otherwise, it is difficult to understand how they could have permitted publication of such unwarranted opinions regarding plant enzymes.

Challenging the wholesomeness of plant enzymes in the animal organism is equivalent to challenging the organism's own economy since all animals bodies manufacture most, if not all of the enzymes found in plants. Oxidase, peroxidase, catalase, amylase, protease, lipase, sucrase, maltase, and numerous other enzymes are found in both animal and plant tissues. To say that these enzymes may not be wholesome in the animal body is an incongruity. I do not deny that plant enzymes rapidly change the color and flavor of vegetables when these are bruised or macerated. Rather it is a difficulty that chemists in the canning industry must contend with. When lipase splits fats in the intestine, the resulting products have a bitter flavor, but that cannot be accepted as an indication that lipase is unwholesome.

Another celebrated advocate of heat-treatment, as applied to milk, is E.V. McCollum, Johns Hopkins University. McCollum's stand is justified to the extent that he chooses what appears (at least as an immediate expedient) to be the lesser of two evils. He appears to be willing to sacrifice an inherent virtue of raw milk in favor of the safety value of pasteurized milk. In one of his publications on the subject, McCollum (330) recites the greater incidence of diphtheria, scarlet fever, and other diseases among 3,700 children, divided into two groups and fed raw milk and heated milk to supplement their diets. The average weight and height of individuals in the two groups was:

	Weight	Height
On raw milk	32.2 LB	37.4"
On pasteurized milk	33.6 LB	37.5"

It is difficult to account for these figures unless it is assumed that there are casual influences attributable to other factors than the milk consumed. Since the results of the survey, as they relate to the weight and height of the children, are totally at variance with other evidence I am about to present, it appears that the assumption of a casual relationship is probably correct. Furthermore, the 3,700 records were collected from 39 cities in 10 states. Larger cities employ pasteurization; many towns and villages do not. Therefore the records of children using pasteurized milk came from cities while those using raw milk came from rural communities. In many respects the diet of rural and urban communities differs. In cities, the consumption of refined carbohydrates by children is greater, and it is altogether probable that the slightly increased growth recorded in this survey is to be attributed to some such stimulation or extraneous influence and not to the milk at all. Certainly, the figures revealed by the survey cannot be shown to deserve any credence since the conditions were equivocal.

McCollum upholds the use of pasteurized milk in these words: "The idea of splitting hairs over slight assumed differences is absurd. It seems strange indeed that when we accept so generally the cooking of most of our foods, there should still remain in certain areas a serious objection to the milk heat treatment involved in pasteurization. Universal pasteurization would be imperative if only for the prevention of the spread of bovine tuberculosis among children". It is not my position here to advocate a practicable diet but rather an optimal one. Obviously, it is not feasible to use commercial raw milk as a food because of its danger as a carrier of disease. But the point at issue is whether raw milk, used as food, can furnish something to the organism, aside from vitamins, not supplied by pasteurized milk.

McCollum and others hold that the effect of pasteurization on the food value of milk is negligible. The considerable destruction of vitamin C it is said, can be compensated for by use of fruit juice. But the lack of this vitamin in the nutrition of the rat is generally considered to be without effect. Thus the point can be easily made that the *only material difference between raw milk and pasteurized milk is that raw milk has a complement of at least half a dozen enzymes* whereas these enzymes are killed to the extent of 85 to 95 per cent or more during pasteurization (331). Consequently, any differences in the health, physical condition, or life span of animals or human beings reared upon raw milk or pasteurized milk can only be ascribed to the influence of the enzymes contained in raw milk.

The comparative effects of raw human milk and pasteurized cows' milk have been studied from birth to 9 months of age in 20,061 babies by Grulee, Sanford, and Herron (332), Rush Medical College. 48.5 per cent were entirely breast-fed, 43 per cent partially breast-fed and 8.5

per cent artificially fed. Total morbidity for the breast-fed infants was 37.4 per cent; for the partially breast-fed 53.8 per cent; and for the artificially fed 63.6 per cent. *Total mortality was 1.1 per cent and, of this, 6.7 per cent was in the breast-fed group, 27.2 per cent in the partially breast-fed, and 66.1 per cent in the artificially-fed group.* Attention must be called to the fact that breast-fed infants received raw milk, while artificially-fed infants were fed on pasteurized milk. It is fairly obvious that if the results of this experiment are appraised simultaneously with all of the other facts linking food enzymes with human welfare, at least some of the superior status of the breast-fed infants must be attributed to the ingested enzymes in the milk.

A survey by Glazier (333) in the Boston area led him to believe that poor development, infection, deficiency diseases, and gastrointestinal diseases are much more frequent in bottle-fed infants than in suckling infants. Mortality was only 1/5 to 1/3 that of bottle-fed babies, and the *breast-fed babies were ill only 1/4 the length of time of the bottle-fed.*

Ederton (334) reported the Lanarkshire Milk Experiment, in which 5,000 children were given 3/4 pint of raw milk a day and 5,000 children in these same schools selected as controls. In another set of schools, 5,000 children were given 3/4 pint of pasteurized milk and another 5,000 children in these same schools were selected as controls. Raw milk was proven superior to pasteurized milk in promoting growth in stature of girls, but no such difference could be demonstrated in boys.

Sprawsen (335), London Hospital, observed that raw milk had specific effect on the teeth of man, conferring considerable immunity to dental caries. It excelled pasteurized and sterilized milk in body-building properties. No incidence of dental caries showed in 40 children brought up on raw milk from the age of $4^1/2$ months to an average age of 4 years, although they had been on diets rich in refined carbohydrates.

Catel (336,337), University Pediatric Clinic, Leipzig, fed 6 premature infants raw human milk for 16 days and they flourished exceedingly well. Then they were transferred to human milk heated at 100°C for 15 minutes, for a period of 16 days or for as long a period as the infants could stand it. On sterilized human milk the rate of growth decreased, diarrhea developed, and there was a catarrhal condition of the respiratory tract and impaired utilization of protein and other materials.

Lasby and Palmer (338) found that the bones of rats fed on raw milk had a slightly higher percentage of ash and a slightly higher content of calcium and phosphorus than the bones of rats fed on pasteurized milk.

Raw or sterilized milk and biscuit of white flour supplemented with Fe, Cu, and Mn were fed to groups of young rats for periods up to 48 weeks by Channon and Channon (339). Samples of milk sterilized by two different processes were compared with the corresponding raw milks drawn from the same bulk samples. After 48 weeks, the weights of the sterilized milk groups were about 10% lower than those of the raw milk groups.

Potter (340) reviewed the therapeutic efficiency attributed to milk in tuberculosis, gastric ulcer, and many other diseases in ancient as well as more recent times. In his own experience comprising several thousand cases on exclusive milk diet, he observed that pasteurized milk was not the equal of raw milk in the realm of therapy. It is obvious that physicians no longer expect much aid from present day pasteurized milk as a remedial agent. Its time honored value as a distinct aid in tuberculosis seems to have vanished with the advent of pasteurization.

During the past 15 years, I have observed something like 200 individuals on diets in which more than 90 per cent of the calorie value was furnished by milk. The diets were continued, as a rule, for periods of one week to two months. These individuals were advised to use certified raw milk, if possible, but many of them found this impracticable and had to resort to pasteurized milk. I have often been able to notice a difference in the reaction of the organism to the two kinds of milk. On pasteurized milk, nasopharyngeal congestion often made an appearance, but not on certified raw milk. Colitis responded better to raw milk. In certain systemic skin afflictions, the lesions frequently disappeared but no such result followed when pasteurized milk was used. At the start of my career as a practitioner, before I evolved the doctrine of food enzymes in relation to nutrition, I used to prescribe raw diets, including raw milk diet and orange diet, by the simple logic that since pasteurization, for instance, was effective in destroying germ life, there should be no good reason why it could not destroy valuable life-like principles in food.

There has been much discussion among so-called food faddists about "live" food, it having been realized that cooked food is no longer "live". There is a discernible undercurrent of opinion among practicing medical men that a certain amount of raw, uncooked food in the diet is indispensable to the highest degree of health. Assuming that the proteins, fats, carbohydrates, minerals, and vitamins are equally available for nutrition in raw and cooked food, any demonstrable nutritional superiority of raw food must then be ascribed to the "live" quality of raw food, and when this live quality is subjected to analysis, it is shown to consist of, or be possessed of, no other property than that possessed by enzymes. The poor showing made on experimental pasteurized milk diets cannot be assigned to vitamin C deficiency, because rats, which are ordinarily used, are not sensitive to sub-normal vitamin C content of food.

Metchnikoff attributed the relatively long life span and freedom from disease of Bulgarian peasants to their consumption of sour milk containing a lactic acid bacillus. The principle of changing the intestinal flora has since found a certain limited applicability. However, Metchnikoff's assumption took no account of a far better explanation. Dairy products form a large proportion of the diet in certain countries. Before the era of pasteurization, dairy products were utilized in the raw condition, since their palatability does not improve by heat-treatment, as is the case with many food materials. When a large share of the calorie requirements was supplied by raw milk, raw butter, and raw cheese, not only did the organism receive a daily quota of enzymes, but the enzyme content of the tissues was not so heavily drawn upon as in those countries where the preponderance of the diet consisted of heat-treated foods. Therefore, the *Bulgarian peasants, many of whom Metchnikoff found to live to the century mark in their mountainous abode, might be expected to have a long life span by virtue of the fact that their enzyme reserve is more slowly used up during the course of living.* That this is the correct explanation can hardly be doubted, since it agrees with facts arrived at experimentally under controlled conditions.

Mattick and Golding (341), National Institute of Dairying Research, University of Reading, fed 3 groups of rats from 7 litters entirely on either raw, pasteurized or sterilized milk with addition of dry flour and water biscuit in each case. Excluding the original rats, 5 generations were obtained in the raw milk group, 3 in the pasteurized, and none in the sterilized milk groups. In the raw and pasteurized groups, the average weights were higher than in the sterilized group, and in the 3rd generations, but not in the original and 2nd generations, the average weights were higher in the raw milk than in the pasteurized milk group. Loss of hair was observed in some rats of the 2nd and 3rd generations of the pasteurized group. The bones of 2nd generation rats of the pasteurized group contained slightly less Ca and total ash than those of 2nd generation raw milk rats. In a final experiment, 2 groups, each of 18 rats, from 7 litters, were given diets of biscuit with raw or pasteurized milk. In the 2nd generation there was no significant difference in the weights of the two groups, but in the 3rd generations the rats on the heated milk were abnormally small. In the heated milk group (but not in the raw milk group), loss of hair occurred in the 2nd and 3rd generations. The hemoglobin content of the blood of 2nd generation rats was slightly higher in the raw milk than in the heated milk rats.

An unbiased study of the influence of pasteurization on the nutritional value of milk was published by Elvehjem and Hart, Dept. of Agricultural Chemistry, and Jackson and Weckel, Dept. of Dairy Industry, University of Wisconsin (342). Raw or pasteurized milk, supplemented with iron, copper, and manganese, was fed as the sole diet to groups of rats at different seasons. The results are tabulated:

AVERAGE DAILY GAINS IN GRAMS DURING
THE FIRST SIX WEEKS

Time of starting Experiment	Raw milk Males	Females	Pasteurized milk Males	Females
October 26, 1932	4.55	3.04	4.36	3.04
April 21, 1933	4.00	2.66	3.49	1.91
October 14, 1933	4.19	2.88	3.90	2.59
December 27, 1933	3.32	2.11	1.96	2.52
February 6, 1934.	2.45	3.14	1.14	2.12

It is seen that pasteurization exerted a markedly detrimental effect on the nutritive value of milk, while milk produced at a time of the year when the cow is receiving an abundance of green feed containing certain essential factors is not effected to the same extent. I quote from the original paper of Elvehjem and his associates: "Some of the reported work on the question of whether pasteurized milk is equal nutritionally to raw milk is valueless because it was sponsored by parties either opposed to or in favor of pasteurized milk. Lack of vitamin C cannot be held accountable for the difference, because rats do no require this factor in the diet. There is no indication that our rats were receiving a limited supply of vitamin A or Vitamins B and G".

A remarkable set of experiments was performed in Japan to test the ability of milk heated at various temperatures to sustain growth and life in young mice. Okada and Sano (343), Biochemical Dept., Government Institute for Infectious Diseases, Tokyo Imperial University, fed groups of mice raw milk and milk heated for 30 minutes at 60, 80, 100, 120, and 140°C. Ten mice were used for each experiment, and the average values showed that the weight of mice fed on milk heated at 60 degrees was 20 per cent less than those fed on raw milk after a seven week period of feeding. Heating at 80 degrees for 30 minutes showed gain in weight at first and then loss, followed by death in 3 weeks.

Heating at 80°C caused death in 3 weeks.
Heating at 100°C caused death in 2 weeks.
Heating at 120°C caused death in 1 week.
Heating at 140°C caused death in 3 to 5 days.

Growth was greatly retarded in rats fed milk heated at higher temperatures.

Arthus (344) found a supplement of fresh milk added to basal diets which produced only moderate growth in young rats, had a remarkable growth-promoting effect, whilst an equivalent supplement of casein had no such effect. These results indicated that milk contains a growth-promoting principle which is not stable to heat, since the growth-promoting effect of milk diminishes progressively with duration of heating at 100°C. The growth-promoting principle differs from vitamin B in being much less resistant to heat, being slowly destroyed even at 60 to 70°C. Furthermore, foods containing vitamin B in abundance did not promote growth in rats if the vital principle was absent. Rats receiving diets composed of dried powdered milk containing the principle, malt extract, flour, and sugar, grew normally; but if the growth-promoting principle of the diet was destroyed by heat, they died, exhibiting symptoms of protein starvation. *It will be noted that the sensitiveness of the growth-promoting substance to heat identifies it at once with enzymes* which are killed at the very temperatures Arthus and the Japanese investigators found to be destructive to the life-supporting and growth-promoting principle in milk.

Chapter 19

THERMO-LABILE SUPPLEMENTARY FACTORS IN MEAT

Fish were fed on raw and cooked meat by Richet and Richard (345) for 205 days and weighed at 10 day intervals. The results on 6 individuals of *Cantharus griseus* were uniformly in favor of raw meat.

McCay and associates (309), in experiments on trout, found that the factor of raw liver which is responsible for the maintenance of life in trout is not identical with any of the known vitamins. When extracts of raw liver were heated at 65°C, they failed to promote growth.

The biologic value of raw beef muscle when fed to rats at the 7 per cent level by Morgan and Kern (346) was greater than that of the same meat cooked in 3 different ways. There appeared to be a heat injury which increased with severity of heat exposure. One portion of the meat, cut into 2 inch cubes, was boiled in water until the internal temperature was 84°C, previous work by these investigators having shown that meat is thoroughly cooked at 84°C. A second portion of the meat cubes was autoclaved at 15 pound pressure until the internal temperature became 84°C, which required 7 minutes. The last portion was autoclaved at 15 pounds for one hour. Raw meat and cooked meat, including the cooking water, were dried at low temperature and fed to rats in powder form, supplemented by fat, cornstarch, agar, salt mixture, and vitamins, with the following results:

	Number of rats	Average Body Initial	Weights Final	Total Food Eaten	Gain in Wt.Per gm of protein Consumed
	gm	gm	gm	gm	
Raw	17	58	126	394	2.58
Boiled	18	58	117	345	2.41
Autoclaved 7 Min.	18	57	118	352	2.44
Autoclaved 1 Hr	18	58	104	356	1.80

Morgan and Kern also noted that when protein is fed at a higher level, the extra protein may make it more difficult or impossible to detect heat injury in short experiments.

It can be realized that the heat injury reported in the three preceding investigations could not have been due to damage to vitamins, since the degree of temperature used (60 to 70°C, 65°C and 84°C), while capable of killing enzymes completely, has been stated to harm vitamins only slightly.

If any doubt exists as to the utter lack of defense of enzymes against destruction by mild heat, I can supply proof, based on my own experiments, as well as those of more than 50 technical men and physicians, that enzymes, if heated in water, are destroyed more or less completely in the temperature range from 48 to 65°C. *Long heating at 48°C or short heating at 65°C kills enzymes. Heating at 60 to 80°C for 1/2 hour completely kills any enzyme.*

There can be little doubt that, except for a few industrial chemists and research investigators who are thrown into intimate contact with the problem, the majority of technical men have only a vague conception of the extreme thermo-lability of enzymes. In United States Department of Agriculture Bulletin No. 342, appears this statement:

"The question whether pasteurization destroys beneficial enzymes is still open. In the light of our present knowledge of the enzymes in milk and the part they play in the digestive process, it is quite impossible to settle the question of their importance. It is evident, however, that the low temperatures now in use in pasteurization have little effect on the commonly recognized enzymes". This was evidently written in 1916, at which time knowledge along these lines was in a rudimentary state. Yet, the bulletin was revised in 1932 and the statement was permitted to stand. The assertion that the low temperatures now in use in pasteurization have little effect on enzymes is not true, since enzymes begin to be destroyed at 48°C (118 degrees F), while the pasteurization temperature is 145 degrees F.

At least half a dozen tests have been proposed, based on the percentage of destruction of enzymes in milk, to check the thoroughness of dairy pasteurization. A series of lectures was recently given on enzymes by the biochemistry department of a well-known university. The lecturer, a competent biochemist, was asked how much heat enzymes can withstand. He answered that very little is known on the subject, but, as an off-hand opinion, he thought they would not survive boiling temperatures. Regardless of how universal such opinions may be, I am, nevertheless, prepared to go into the subject in detail and show there is complete unanimity of opinion among those having first hand knowledge of the subject, on the extreme sensitivity of enzymes to heat.

Chapter 20

DIET AND HEALTH OF PRIMITIVE
AND MODERNIZED ESKIMOS

It must be brought out that most savage and primitive races, with the exception of the isolated Eskimo, utilize cookery. *The primitive, isolated polar Eskimo is perhaps the only primitive type not having the medicine man as an official member of the tribe with a full complement of remedies.* It is true, they have their witch doctors, but these act mostly in the capacity of spiritual leaders, although it is said they have been known to do crude but skillful surgery in instances of injury. However, it appears that the primitive Eskimo has had neither the urge nor the necessity to develop the art of preparing and using substances as medicines.

The excellent health of the primitive Eskimo is stated by a number of qualified observers to be surpassed by no other race of people on this earth and equaled by few if any. And this in spite of the fact that the Eskimo diet is composed principally of meat and fish, which is usually regarded as unfavorable and not conducive to maximum health. I am sure that nearly every physician would regard the great consumption of flesh foods by the Eskimo (reputed to amount to more than 10 pounds per day in times of plenty) as burdensome if not calamitous. But the *meat is consumed usually and preferably raw,* and I believe it is not necessary at this stage of the writing, in view of what has been presented so far, to stress acceptance of the doctrine that it is by virtue of the fact that the Eskimo eats a large share of his food raw that he is enabled to display such high health standards. The Eskimo, like the wild animal, partakes much of his food in the natural state, with all of the original enzymes intact.

On the other hand, cooking tribes, such as the American Indian or jungle peoples, have had a more or less comprehensive materia medica, composed of a variety of substances mostly of vegetable or animal origin. Among these tribes, the urge to use medicines appears to be strong. It is interesting to note that the appearance of a systematic materia medica is correlated with the practice of extensive cookery among these peoples. An otherwise healthful outdoor life does not prevent onset of certain diseases. Instances of arthritis appearing among primitive red men, as well as in their ancient skeletal remains, have been reported. There are, therefore, excellent reasons for the contention that these diseases have a nutritional origin. Since primitives do not refine their flour, peel fruit or vegetables, or use concentrated or refined foods, such as sugar, it cannot be argued that there can be any significant vitamin or mineral deficiency. But the practice of cookery engenders an enzyme-deficient diet which is thus left as the sole explanation for diseases in otherwise healthful surroundings.

Everyone acquainted with the application of therapeutic diets has had occasion to witness the beneficial effects often following use of the raw diet in one form or another. The benefits following the Salisbury diet might be conveniently explained as due to use of rare meat, the inner portion of which is raw and possessed of its natural enzymes. Potter's raw milk diet had found wide therapeutic use during the time when milk was generally available in the raw form. The healthful and therapeutic virtues of various forms of raw grape, raw apple, raw orange, and raw vegetable diet are thoroughly appreciated by those having experience in their use.

Dr. Thomas (347), physician for the Macmillan Arctic Expedition, found that the Greenland Eskimo, on a carnivorous diet, ate his food usually and preferably raw and exhibited no increased tendency to vascular or renal disease, scurvy, or rickets, while the Labrador Eskimo, whose meat was cooked and whose diet included many prepared, dried, and canned articles, is very much subject to scurvy and rickets. The diet of the Greenland Eskimo includes the meat of whale, walrus, seal, caribou, musk ox, Arctic hare, polar bear, fox, ptarmigan, and the numerous sea gulls, geese, duck, auks, gulls, and also fish, all eaten usually and preferably raw. Blubber is used in lighting and warming the domiciles, in melting ice and snow for drinking, and to a much lesser extent in cooking food.

As a member of the Putnam Baffin Island Expedition, Heinbecker, (348), Departments of Biological Chemistry and Physiology, Washington University School of Medicine, visited Baffin Island Eskimos and studied their blood and urine chemistry. All of the urine specimens were free from sugar. The Eskimos showed no ketosis, having a remarkable power to oxidize fats completely, as evidenced by the small amount of acetone bodies excreted in the urine during fasting. It is well known that in most human subjects ketosis appears when the material metabolized is restricted to protein and fat. According to Shaffer's (349) analysis, the metabolism of the foodstuffs contained in the Eskimo diet produces ketosis when fed to human beings in the temperate zones. The Eskimo, being on a high-protein diet, containing considerable seal fat, should be subject to ketosis, other things being equal. However, if the food is consumed raw, a profound influence is introduced. After feeding Caspian seal fat to experimental animals for 5 to 9 months, Nephriakhin and Berezin (350) observed that the lipase content in blood and organs showed a small, yet stable and definite increase. Lipase has been found more or less concentrated in many raw, natural fats. It is not unlikely that freedom of the Eskimo from ketosis is related to ingestion of lipase with the food, causing better metabolism of fat than is the case with persons subsisting on the conventional heat-treated diet. Heinbecker observed that most fresh meat was eaten partly boiled and the remainder raw. Frozen meat was generally eaten raw. When food of any type was cached for some time and became "high" (autolyzed), it was eaten raw.

Garber (351) lived a number of years among Eskimos in Northern Alaska and had occasion to observe their habits. Quotation: "Fish are put into a hoe and covered with grass and earth and the mass is allowed to ferment and decay. I learned, to my utter astonishment, that they would eat those rotten, poisonous foods and thrive on them. Lest the reader might think that the cooking process would destroy the poisons in their vitiated foods, I wish to say that in only a few instances did they cook their food. The usual and customary method was to devour it raw".

Price (352) visited the Alaskan Eskimo to determine the *incidence of caries* and found the number of teeth involved in caries for each 1,000 teeth examined was *0.9 for the primitive Eskimo and 130 for the modernized Eskimo.*

Urquhart (353), a physician practicing among the Eskimos of Northern Canada near Aklavik, has never seen a single case of malignancy during 7 years of practice in the region. Gastric or duodenal ulcer, acute or chronic nephritis, or scurvy, are extremely rare. Teeth are in excellent condition. Rheumatic fever, asthma, and the common cold are rare. In the performance of urinalyses running well into the thousands during seven years, not a single case of glycosuria was seen. Fish fills a large part of their menu and they eat the entire fish raw and very "high".

Stefansson (2) lived with Eskimos in the Mackenzie River District for a number of years and reported conclusive evidence of a high degree of average good health and no incidence of caries, scurvy, rickets, or cancer. When meat is cooked, chunks of the frozen meat, varying in size from that of a lemon to that of a grapefruit, are heated in water over a small flame until boiling commences. Under these conditions of cookery it is doubtful if the internal temperature becomes high enough to be destructive to enzymes. Stefansson states that Eskimo custom ordains that the inside of each piece shall be rare. It is thus quite probable that even in the cooked meat some of the enzymes are preserved.

Rabinowitch (354,355), Department of Metabolism, Montreal General Hospital, visited Eskimos in Hudson Bay and Strait, Baffin Island, Devon, and Ellesmere Islands, as a member of the Canadian Government Eastern Arctic Patrol on the *R.M.S. Nascopie*. The purpose was to compile official information on the health of the Eskimo with the idea of preventing extinction of the race. The following is quoted from Rabinowitch's reports: "In all, 389 were examined. The use of flour was found to be determined by the availability of meat. In Hudson's Bay, for example, at Chesterfield Inlet, hunting conditions are poor and flour was very common; it was found in 8 of 19 tents visited. Whereas, in the same Bay, at Coral Harbor on Southampton Island, where seal hunting is good near the Post, flour was found in only 1 of 8 tents visited. At Lake Harbour, with good hunting, flour was found in only 1 of 26 tents. Whereas at Port Burwell, where hunting is poor, flour was found in all of the 9 tents visited. Tuberculosis was common in the Straits and Bay (Chesterfield Inlet). No evidence of the disease was found at Clyde River, Pont Inlet and Dundas Harbour on Devon Island. The teeth very strikingly differentiate the Eskimo of the Straits and Bay from those of the more northerly regions. In the Bay and Straits many were quite clean, and the reason was obvious; they had been brushed. However the highest incidence of caries and pyorrhea was found in this region. Of 31 natives examined, 16 had very poor teeth. As we traveled north, the teeth were found in a much filthier state, but they were much healthier. In the matter of arteriosclerosis, the Bay and Straits again differ from the more northerly regions. Thickened radial and tortuous temporal vessels were common, and in 34 cases the blood pressures were greater than 150 mm Hg. No evidence of arteriosclerosis was found at Clyde River, Pond Inlet, Dundas, and Craig Harbor. Of 39 films taken in Hudson's Bay and Straits, 19 showed definite calcification of the arteries, whereas of 24 films on Baffin Island, 4 only showed calcification, in spite of the fact that the average age of the Hudson and Straight group was 44.6 years against 50 years for the Eskimos in Hudson's Bay and Straits and 38 in the more northerly regions. In all 9 had albuminuria and all, with one exception, were from Hudson's Bay and Straits. When food is abundant, a healthy Eskimo, living under primitive conditions, will eat 5 to 10 pounds of meat or more a day and the greatest meat eaters are in the northerly regions. The Eskimo disturbs our ideas about high-protein diet. There were no signs of any heart disease except an apical murmur in one case. All of the tonsils had healthy pink surfaces and no pus was found upon pressure. No case of cancer or diabetes mellitus was seen and of all urine examined only 3 cases contained reducing substances, but these were subsequently found to be non-fermentable. Nor were there any acetone bodies in any of the urines".

Chapter 21

THERAPEUTIC VALUE OF RAW FOOD DIETS

The *therapeutic value of raw diets is clearly recognized by many physicians.* Generally, the principle is utilized by increasing the consumption of fruits and vegetables which are palatable in the natural, raw state, and decreasing the amount of heat-treated, high calorie foods. I have found, however, that the same results are attainable in many instances without decreasing the calorie value of the diet, by replacing the heat-treated, high-calorie foods with palatable raw foods of substantially equal calorie value. In this connection, use can often be made of unheated honey, raw egg yolk, unpasteurized milk, raw butter, raw cheese, thoroughly ripe banana, avocado, dates and figs, and sometimes tree nuts in the shell. I have found exclusive use of orange juice in many diseases accompanied by fever, shortens the duration and mitigates the severity of the condition. This is especially true of many of the exanthematous diseases of childhood. Canned orange juice or canned tomato juice is not conducive to the same decisive improvement.

In gastric disease and colitis, the raw milk diet has been of unquestionable value. In hypertension, I have seen reduction in the systolic blood pressure ranging up to more than 75 mm through use of properly planned diets consisting mainly of raw food. Close to 500 of these hypertension cases have come under my observation and, even in the long-term cases, considerable reductions, accompanied by appropriate symptomatic improvement, were secured when the individual would adhere to the regimen for a sufficient period. Chronic arthritis requires long continued effort, but the lessened pain and improved joint movement are undeniable evidences of what a raw food diet can accomplish if designed to sustain the weight and vitality at a proper level. Many cases of various neuralgic conditions have responded to orange diet used intermittently with raw food diet. Certain types of dysmenorrhea and a host of other maladies frequently met with have likewise been successfully dealt with. I pursue the policy of believing that these therapeutic properties of raw food are due largely, if not entirely, to its enzyme content. I have noticed that canned orange or tomato juices do not achieve the same success as the raw article and that pasteurized milk does not serve the therapeutic role of raw milk.

The German literature is prolific in substantiating the therapeutic properties of raw food. In a study of the food habits of different peoples, King, Kugelmass, and Boedecker (356) observed that "a constant characteristic of all dietaries of races immune to caries is the minimal interference with food as obtained in its natural state. The greater portion of the food consumed, whatever it may be, is necessarily raw, or, at the most, steamed. Cooking of food in primitive races as compared with civilized races, parallels, in a sense, the minimal and extreme incidence of caries".

In this connection, it might be emphasized that destruction of enzymes by heat requires that they be subjected to the influence of moist heat. For instance, it has been shown that heating powdered pancreatin or malt amylase to 100°C does not result in material damage. Dry heat is not destructive except when the temperature is raised to 150°C. When foods are merely steamed in a primitive manner, it is questionable as to how much destruction of enzymes occurs. While the destruction in cookery with modern highly efficient equipment is 100 per cent, steaming with crude utensils may result in only a partial loss.

Loewy and Behrens (357) point out that although *raw diets are of therapeutic value in certain gastrointestinal disorders, renal diseases, hypertension, diabetes, gout, some forms of obesity, and in many skin diseases,* they are not, however, to be considered the normal diets for healthy persons. An addition of cooked food is desirable for most persons.

According to Glassner (358), a diet consisting of uncooked vegetables, fruits, and nuts is useful in the treatment of a variety of conditions such as acute and chronic nephritis, obesity, gastrointestinal disorders, and certain heart conditions. Certain diseases of the skin, especially those of an allergic nature, for example urticaria and eczema, respond to it, and it is also valuable in treatment of tuberculosis of the skin.

Eimer (359) used food of vegetable origin, untouched by any cooking process, in the management of renal or cardiac edema; in diseases of the circulatory system, in high blood pressure and in diabetes, with good results. It aided peristalsis and did not cause gastric disturbance in healthy persons.

The modern raw diet regime is of value in certain avitaminosis, nephritis, diabetes, cardiac disease, and chronic constipation (360).

Just (361) reported employment of 3 types of predominantly raw diets in his German sanitarium. First, uncooked fruit exclusively; second, uncooked fruit and uncooked vegetables; third, uncooked fruit and uncooked vegetables with additions of rye, vita-type bread, cereals, milk, and milk products and, occasionally, raw eggs. The first and second types are for short periods only, although the second may be continued for several weeks. The third type may be taken permanently if desired. Fruit and raw vegetable diet is indicated in diseases of metabolism and of the heart and blood vessels; in disorders involving the internal secretions; in hypovitaminosis; in diseases of the blood vessels and nerves; and in fevers. The diet is contraindicated in pernicious anemia and other blood diseases; in organic nervous diseases; in severe pulmonary tuberculosis; and in many nervous and mental diseases.

In his sanitarium in Switzerland, Bircher-Benner (362,363) claims to have attained a large measure of success with the raw food regime in diabetes, ulcer, Graves' disease, arthritis, asthma, and other conditions not commonly attributed to faulty nutrition. Bircher-Benner ascribes great value to raw food because it contains vital properties that he calls "light accumulators". Dr. Bircher-Benner is evidently trying to find a cause for observed effects. But it is not necessary to invent new food entities, since those now known, namely enzymes, can explain all of the observed therapeutic phenomena and, furthermore can be subjected to fairly rigid scientific scrutiny, which is not yet the case with hypothetical entities such as Dr. Bircher-Benner's 'light accumulators'. Enzymes are profoundly influenced by light, according to the limited amount of experimental data available.

Quoting Dr. Bircher-Benner: "There are two kinds of human health. True health, such as one rarely sees nowadays, and the appearance of health, which I would like to call 'pregnant ill health.' What we have been pleased to call 'good health,' is, in reality, a very long incubation period preceding the appearance of active disease. I arranged the materials of human nutrition into three classes according to their values as light accumulators:

CLASS 1- *Raw plant organs and products: nuts, oil, honey; milk from healthy and rightly-nourished cows. Possibly, also raw eggs from healthy and rightly fed hens.*
CLASS 2- Wholemeal bread; rightly-prepared and cooked vegetable food; cooked milk and dairy produce; cooked eggs.
CLASS 3- All kinds of meat dishes, canned and preserved food, white flour products, refined sugar, mushrooms, etc.

The more severe, obstinate, and constitutional the illness, the more must nutrition belonging to the first class of light accumulators preponderate".

Bircher-Benner continues: "Gurwitsch, a Russian, has now proved incontrovertibly that the living substance does actually fluoresce. Thus, ultra-violet rays are emitted from a raw onion, whilst in one that is cooked they are extinguished. Lakhovsky, a physicist living in Paris, says in his book, *The Mystery of Life*, that living cells contain highly-charged molecules and 'combined formations" he calls them 'biomagnomobiles,' which are of the greatest importance to life and can be replaced only through raw food. *The exclusion of raw food from human diet since the bacteriological era, he thinks, brought about terrible consequences, particularly the increase of cancer.* Lakhovsky calls cancer the price which humanity pays for asepsis".

Hackh (364), College of Physicians and Surgeons, San Francisco, writing of the influence of enzymes on life processes, remarked: "The most fundamental reactions occurring in living protoplasm are hydration and dehydration. The formation of water and its liberation is the most significant reaction in the synthesis and decomposition of proteins, fats, and carbohydrates. Building starch from sugar, proteins from amino-acids, fats from acids and alcohols, the reaction proceeds from left to right; in the decomposition of carbohydrates, proteins, and fats, it proceeds from right to left. Whichever way the reaction goes, we need certain substances, the enzymes, and perhaps vitamins, which apparently control the direction and speed of these reactions. Should these reactions stop, then paraplasm is formed, or the protoplasm is degenerated and dead. What mechanism can be suggested to keep the molecules and atoms on the move? Let us answer 'Light.' Light is being constantly absorbed by growing plants. It is necessary in the animal body to activate the reactions in the animal body. Light energy is being constantly lost by radiation, for protoplasm emits a faint fluorescence, hence must be replaced to keep protoplasm alive, which may come through 'living' food like fresh, raw vegetables and fruits, and through exposure to light".

The allegations of the two preceding accounts may be properly adjudged by comparison with the material of this manuscript. I include them here to show that the *value of the thermo-labile principles in raw food is being repeatedly observed by individuals in the medical profession*, and that *there is a persistent effort to valuate the labile principle of* "live" *food in terms of vital energy. Unless the role of food enzymes in life processes is clearly perceived, such effort is likely to be poorly directed.*

I believe Copiscarow (365,366) has clearly shown that metabolic ultra-violet rays, or so-called biological fluorescence, is due to enzymic activity. He wrote as follows: "In the current issue of 'Protoplasma' (21:73, 1934), I brought forward experimental evidence which leaves no doubt that metabolic ultra-violet radiation (Gurwitsch or Mitogenetic rays) finds its source in the activity of oxidation enzymes. It thus appears that the function of oxidation enzymes represents a combination of the contact phase (carbohydrate, phosphorus and sulfur metabolism) with that of induction, responsible for cell mitosis, chromosome modifications, and gene mutations - the two phases of enzyme activity being complementary to one another. In the case of metabolic radiations in the visible spectrum range, we find phosphorescence or bio-luminescence to be exhibited by various types of bacteria, oceanic micro-organisms, fungi, mollusc pholas, glowing sea worms, glow worm, fire fly, and probably higher organisms. From the work of Beijerink and Harvey, Hajasi, and Okuyama, and Warburg and Christian, (references given) it appears that this *bio-luminescence is a function of oxidation enzymes"*.

Protti (367) measured the ultra-violet radiation of the blood and correlated it with enzymic activity. He claimed that the radiant power of the blood is a physico-chemical property manifested by emission of electro-magnetic radiation belonging to the ultra-violet field. This photo-electric manifestation is closely associated with processes of combustion of polypeptides and carbohydrates. Previous experimental data by Protti support the view that the radiant power of blood is an index of the oxidative and enzymic process occurring in the organism. Blood radiometric results are discussed in relation to age groups, sex, diet, etc. The average inductive effect of male and female bloods is #44.4. Bloods are classified according to their radiant power as:

SUBRADIANT   0 to 30
AVERAGE   35 to 60
SUPERRADIANT   50 to 90

Blood radiometric data seem to support the hypothesis that equal radiometric figures correspond to equal or equivalent metabolic rhythms.

At the International Canine Congress, Monaco, in 1934 (368), 11 papers were presented by experts from 8 countries. The following is a summary of conclusions: "The feeding of dogs should have as its basis raw meat (by raw meat is meant muscular tissue, bones, viscera, glands, blood, etc.). There may also be included in the diet, biscuits, dry bread, rice, or cereals. These two types of food may be fed in equal quantities". Veterinarians recognize raw meat as indispensable if good physical condition is to be maintained for long periods.

Leven and Butin (369), Central Scientific Institute of Nutrition, Moscow, *recommended* a diet entirely composed of *raw vegetables* for a short period as a treatment for *arthritis*.

Exclusive diets of raw apple and banana have achieved considerable vogue in pediatric practice in treatment of dysentery. As many as 20 apples daily can be used by adults. A prolific literature has developed on the subject.

Sherman (370) maintained rats on a diet consisting of a mixture of 5/6 raw ground whole wheat and 1/6 dried whole milk, with table salt and distilled water. It supported normal growth and health with successful reproduction and rearing of young, generation after generation.

At the Northwestern University Laboratories, Ivy and his associates have frequently maintained dogs for long periods on 3/4 pound of raw lean hamburger and a mixture of a small quantity of bread and milk each day for a 40 pound dog. I mention this to refute the somewhat prevalent notion that raw meat is not good for dogs. There is *ample evidence that free choice is no better a guide for animals than it is for man in proper selection of food.* Free choice may be an effective guide in a choice between natural food materials, unaffected by preparation or heat damage. Given a mixed diet, omnivora and carnivora will invariably choose heat-treated food in preference to raw food. Rats will prefer boiled potato to raw potato, or bread to ground whole wheat. Dogs choose cooked meat first when a choice is to be made between raw and cooked meat. I do not imply that food should be eaten without relish, but only that free choice in a mixed diet is no more trustworthy than is reliance on the senses in use of alcohol, tobacco, or narcotic drugs, assuming, of course, that immoderate use of these substances is open to objection.

Dove (371) studied the nutritive instincts in rat, chick, and dairy calf over a period of years, and found that some individuals were wise and others less wise in their choice of food.

It is incumbent on critical observers to evaluate the special properties of a raw diet, not in terms of vitamins, which are injured relatively little, but in terms of heat labile enzymes which are completely destroyed by ordinary culinary procedures involving use of heat. Some vitamin workers have attempted to justify cookery by pointing out that vitamins are relatively heat stable. *It is just as much an error to measure the value of food by its vitamin content, as it was 30 years ago to judge the useful qualities of food solely by the amounts of protein, carbohydrate, and fat* contained in it. To assume that enzymes of foods are of no value to the body is to repeat the mistake of 50 years ago when it was taken for granted that the so-called ash of foods, which is now known to contain valuable minerals such as calcium and iron, was not needed by the body. Bearing in mind the evidence I have amassed, such an error is now inexcusable.

There is a prevalent notion that persons using much raw food and little prepared protein and carbohydrate foods cannot tolerate high temperatures as well as those following customary diet. Eimer and Kaufmann (372) point out it is generally assumed that since in perspiration not only water, but also sodium chloride is eliminated, the heat regulation of human beings can be adequate only if that which is lost is quickly replaced. That is, in addition to large quantities of fluids, considerable amounts of NaCl (common salt) have to be taken. On the other hand, a person who does not add NaCl to his food, that is, one who lives on a diet that is deficient in NaCl, is supposedly less efficient in hot weather, because he does not have the amount of perspiration necessary for heat regulation. Contrary observations on persons living on a salt-free raw diet induced the authors to make comparative tests on the heat regulation and sweat secretion of persons receiving diets with high, normal, or low NaCl content. It was found that persons on a salt-free raw food diet tolerated the sweating bath generally better than others. The perspiration set in later, the skin and body temperatures did not rise so high, the quantity of perspiration was less, and its percental, as well as absolute NaCl content, was lower. The urine output of Chloride was also lower.

Two young men observed by Stohr (373) took diets containing less than 1 gm of NaCl per day for periods of 36 and 51 days. The urine Cl diminished to low levels. The blood Chloride was high during the experimental period.

Rabinowitch and Smith (355) observed that salt is not used by Eskimos. In 34 Eskimos, the concentration of chlorides in the urine was extremely low. In spite of these low values, chlorides in the plasma were greater than the renal threshold level of NaCl in whites.

Eimer and Voigt (374) described 4 cases of renal disease in which the dehydration and desalination following use of raw food diets (raw vegetables, raw egg, raw milk products) is illustrated. The change does not cease on the second or third day, as in the healthy organism, but continues until the body stores of H_2O and NaCl have been greatly depleted.

Chapter 22

HYPOGLYCEMIC AND HYPOGLYCOSURIC
ACTION OF ENZYMES

The fact that *uncooked foods supply active principles* is illustrated by the work of Rosenthal and Ziegler (375), George Washington University Hospital and Hygienic Laboratory. Fifty grams of raw starch was administered to 7 patients, and 75 grams to another 2 patients, free from alimentary disease or diabetes. Blood sugar showed an average increase of 1 mg per 100 mL in 1/2 hour, a decrease of 1.2 mg in 1 hour, and a decrease of 3 mg in 2 hours. When 50 grams of cooked starch was given the average increase was 56 mg in 1/2 hour; 51 mg in 1 hour, and 11 mg in 2 hours after the meal. Fifty grams of raw starch was eaten by 7 diabetic patients to whom no insulin had been given for several days. Average increase in blood sugar was 6 mg in 1/2 hour, a decrease of 9 mg in 1 hour, and a decrease of 14 mg in 2 1/2 hours after the starch meal. This *fall of blood sugar* below the initial value is worthy of notice. It was negligible in the normal cases, but *in the diabetics* it *varied from 14 to 35 mg.*

Yeast is a good source of certain enzymes, particularly sucrase. Experiments, too numerous to mention, are reported on the hypoglycemic effect of yeast, both in the normal animal and in human diabetes. Bufano (376) prepared extracts of yeast by the Michaelis method and found the extract was in reality a purified invertase solution. Injected into rabbits, it induced more or less uniform decrease in total and free sugar.

Holland and collaborators (377) obtained reductions in blood sugar content in diabetic patients averaging 30 mg per 100 mL by oral administration of 10 egg yolks per individual. The active substance is very labile, attempts to purify it having resulted in the destruction of its hypoglycemic action.

Yeast and enzyme preparations, in addition to enzymes, may contain insuloids, which are heat stable and can cause confusing results when efforts are made to identify active ingredients. Many reports indicate that intravenous or oral administration of amylase exerts hypoglycemic effects in normal and especially in diabetic individuals. That this effect of the enzyme is independent of insuloids is shown by the fact that ligation of pancreatic ducts in rabbits, dogs, and chickens either lowered the blood sugar level or improved the tolerance for carbohydrates.

Reports by Herxheimer [1926], Alpern and Beauglow [1928], Sussi [1930], Nather, Priessel and Wagner [1926], Mansfeld and Szirtes [1928], Ladurner and Unterrichter [1927], Takats [1930], and Ikushima [1930] show the hypoglycemic tendency.

I have already shown that ligation of the pancreatic duct invariably increases the serum amylase level. Thus it is seen that the greater the content of enzyme in the blood, the smaller will be the amount of sugar contained therein, at least within certain limits. Cohen (378) and Reid, Quigley and Myers (261), have proved experimentally on dogs and rabbits that amylase acts to promote storage of sugar in the liver, where, under the influence of insulin, its action becomes reversible to form glycogen from dextrose.

Rosefeld (379,380) noted that injection of amylase resulted in a fall of the blood sugar in normal rabbits and a decrease in the urinary sugar and blood sugar level in diabetic dogs. He concluded that the fall in blood sugar level which follows ligation of the ducts of the salivary glands is due to absorption of amylase from these glands.

The pancreatic digest, obtained by acting upon minced pancreas with fresh pancreatic juice, produced a marked fall of the blood sugar level in 46 cases out of 49, whether it was given by mouth or intravenously, according to the report by Geness and Epstein (381).

Many year ago, Jones (382) noted that oral use of malt amylase decreased the percentage of glucose in the urine of diabetics.

A number of clinicians have discovered that there is a preliminary rise in blood sugar which precedes the decrease consequent to intravenous injection of amylase. Some claim heating the enzyme solution weakens or destroys the sugar-reducing effect; others, that heating has no influence. Evidently, heating abolishes that part of the hypoglycemic effect due to the enzyme, but is without influence on the insuloids.

Reid and Narayana (383) explained that the effects of the intravenous injection of 1 to 2 grams of malt amylase into dogs varied according to whether the animal had been fed recently or had been kept without food for at least two days - the blood sugar level rising in the former case from 0.08 per cent to 0.10 per cent in the course of an hour or two, and falling in the latter from about 0.072 per cent to as low as 0.03 per cent in the course of 3 hours following the injection of amylase.

Deichmann-Grubler and Myers (384) showed that subcutaneous injection of fungus amylase and other amylase preparations into normal persons minimized the hyperglycemic effect resulting from the ingestion of 80 grams of glucose. The glycemic curve was much flatter and the hypoglycemic phase more marked. In diabetes, with a fasting blood sugar level of 160 mg per 100 mL, a favorable effect was observed with 100 to 150 mg of the enzyme and the urinary sugar almost disappeared after 3 hours.

Wilson and Strieck (385) obtained a sharp drop in the blood sugar level of rabbits by intravenous injection of malt amylase. The blood sugar level of a depancreatized dog was similarly affected.

Ottenstein (386) gave diabetic individuals an intravenous injection of malt amylase and observed a fall in the blood sugar level within one to two hours, and a decrease in urine sugar, in one case, from 2 to 0.2 per cent within 3 to 4 hours.

On a salt-poor, high-carbohydrate diet, plus pancreatic extract, 9 unselected patients having old arteriosclerosis with nephritis, aortic disease, or essential hypertension, were clinically observed by Halprin (387). Those who were unable to follow the diet were advised to eat their daily meals and to add 3 oranges or 3 apples to their diet. The pancreatic extract, of which 7 grams were used at each meal, was prepared specially from the fresh (not frozen) gland, without heating and without alcohol extraction. Oral administration of this dried pancreas was shown to lower the blood sugar level in normal individuals. The patients complained of occipital headache, dizziness, spots in front of the eyes, and shortness of breath and after one month had lost 2 to 4 pounds and felt symptomatically better from the regime. Blood pressures invariably showed a drop in the diastolic pressure to below 100. A drop of from 10 to 20 mm in the systolic pressure was shown by 4 patients after 5 months.

Van Steenis (246) presented records to show that the external secretion of the pancreas is often deficient in enzymes in cases of diabetes mellitus. Oral administration of pancreatin, up to 12 grams daily, had a beneficial effect.

Barbera and Adinolfi (249) found enzyme deficiency in the fluids in diabetes which were normalized by administration of raw pancreas, or of a preparation of dried pancreas.

In an extensive experience with diabetes, Bassler (253) reported that over 86 per cent of the cases showed deficiency of amylase in the duodenal contents. Those diabetic individuals showing normal pancreatic juice did well by simple dietetic management without insulin or pancreatic therapy. In the majority, the amylase was diminished and they achieved satisfactory results with diet and pancreatic therapy and without insulin. *At least 50 per cent of the diabetics* who were users of insulin, and in whom the test showed a deficient external secretion of amylase, *could be maintained blood and urine sugar negative on diet and pancreatin alone.*

The literature contains many reports relating to an improvement in the blood sugar level and a decreased excretion of sugar in the urine in diabetes mellitus after ingestion of raw beef pancreas.

The pancreas of fowl, administered orally to diabetic patients by Vannocci (388), resulted in a diminution of sugar in the urine.

Chapter 23

THERAPEUTIC ACTIVITY OF ENZYMES EXTRACTS

Bassler (389), Milliken (390), and Wolffe (391), report *good results* with pancreatic feeding and pancreatic extract in *angina pectoris.*

Remarkable improvement was noted by Walker (392) in 4 cases of *arthritis deformans* through use of a starch-free diet and 30 grains of pancreatin orally per day.

Brown (393) found the pancreatic enzymes in sprue (a chronic disease) to be diminished. Subsequent oral administration of 5 to 10 grains of pancreatin extract 3 times a day was followed by remarkable improvement.

Other reports attesting to the value of raw pancreas or pancreatin in sprue are by Lambert [1923], Castellani [1925,1930], and Silverman [1927].

Fiessinger and Gajdos (394) found subcutaneous injection of liver lipase given to patients with liver cirrhosis had considerable remedial value, and parenteral administration significantly lengthened the life of P-poisoned dogs with ligated pancreatic ducts.

Schweitzer (395) reported success with the use of pancreatin in dermatological practice.

Bodechtel and Kinklin (396) recite experiments by which it had been demonstrated that dried papaya is harmless, well tolerated, and an aid to digestion. They recommend it in achylia, anacidity, dyspepsia, and disorders of the bile passages.

Mostel (397), First Medical Division, General Hospital, Vienna, found prepared Papaya to be of great benefit in digestive disturbances of widely different kinds.

Palombi (398) obtained good results in digestive tract therapy with fungus amylase.

Ivy (273), Dept. of Physiology, Northwestern University Medical School stated: "I suspect that a deficiency of external pancreatic secretion occurs more frequently in man than is now believed. There can be little doubt as to the *oral effectiveness of enzymes administered in the presence of pancreatic deficiency.*"

Animal tissue fat, cream, and olives have been found by a number of investigators to contain sizable quantities of lipase if examined before the materials were subjected to heat treatment. On the other hand it has been reported that in human obesity the lipase content of the fat is decreased. Dell'Acqua (399) found that the lipase content of adipose tissue from cases of human obesity and from lipomas was less than normal.

Raw seal fat was found by Nephriakhin and Berezin (400) to have properties similar to cod liver oil. Fed to rabbits, rats, and guinea pigs over a period of 5 to 9 months, it promoted hematopoiesis. The lipase content in the blood and organs showed a small yet stable and definite increase.

Liver lipase administered subcutaneously by Fiessinger and Gajdos (394) to human patients in liver cirrhosis showed more active healing power than any other medicament. It lengthened the life of P-poisoned dogs with ligated pancreatic ducts.

Virtanen and Soumalainen (17) noted that when large amounts of pig pancreas lipase are subcutaneously injected into guinea pigs, most of the enzyme was retained; the greatest storage occurring in the liver. The same was true of rabbits. The amount of liver lipase could be doubled by injection of pancreatic lipase.

These reports show that *enzymes introduced into the organism are regularly stored in organs and tissues.* They support the contention of Oelgoetz and associates (13) who were able to show that pancreatic extract is stored to the extent of increasing the amylase content of the liver and spleen from 2 to 17 times over the original.

Belkina and Kremlev (401) found that, after injection of catalase in rabbits, the greatest accumulation occurs in the kidneys and muscles.

It is recommended by Messerli (402) that enzymic materials be taken as a regular part of the diet.

Male rats were given 5 mL of raw milk, or a milk and malt mixture, by stomach tube. After one hour, they were killed. Minz and Schilf (403) report that when malt enzymes were added the milk curd was much finer and the degree of digestion much greater than with the milk alone.

Maignon published a series of papers extending from the year 1922 to 1937 (404 to 408 incl.) in which he expostulates upon his doctrine on the remarkable *therapeutic effects of tissue enzymes.* Extracts are made of lungs, stomach, kidney, liver, and other organs by the method of Lebedeff. The extracts behave as biochemical catalysts in prolonged electrolysis and not as inert proteins. They have no effect in normal subjects but show organ specificity when injected into subjects showing insufficiency of liver, kidneys, and other organs. Maignon claims the effect is not due to a hormone but ascribes it to the catalytic action of these enzymes in facilitating the nutrition of the diseased organ. Organ enzyme extracts produced specific effects on the corresponding organ and re-established normal nutrition in subjects with kidney and liver disorders. In aged dogs with renal or hepatic insufficiency as indicated by determination of blood urea and nitrogen, a single injection of 1 mg improved the blood picture. The effect lasted 1 to 2 weeks and 5 to 6 weeks intervened before pre-experimental values returned. A second injection had similar effects. Maignon proved the effects were not due to vitamin B or C, since injection of the tissue enzymes into pigeons suffering from avitaminosis B and into scorbutic guinea pigs failed to influence these conditions.

Turkeltaub and associates (409) fed raw ox heart to patients with heart disease and found improvement in cardiac function and relief of excessive blood pressure.

That improved starch and protein digestion can be attained through use of enzymes even in the normal organism is proved by a number of records to be found in the literature. Hervey (410), working at the New Jersey Agriculture Experiment Station, fed a vegetable fungus enzymic material containing rich concentrations of amylase and protease to four groups of chicks at the rate of 1, 2, 3, and 5 per cent of their mash rations. There were 100 chicks in each of the four groups and 95 in a fifth control group. During 20 weeks feeding, in every instance, the chicks consuming the enzyme material made a more rapid gain in weight than the control chicks. Also, the gain was proportional to the amount of enzyme material eaten. Tests upon the contents of the crop and gizzard at the end of the sixth week of age indicated increased starch and protein digestion in chicks consuming enzymic material over those not consuming it. The final weight, grain, and mash consumption for each bird are given below:

Enzymes Fed %	Number of Chicks	Mean Weight Lb	Mean total Grain eaten Lb	Mean total Mash eaten Lb
5	100	3.24	7.65	8.31
3	100	3.03	7.67	8.31
2	100	2.89	7.68	8.27
1	100	2.80	7.70	8.21
NONE	95	2.65	7.77	7.73

McCandish and Struthers (411) reported that the replacement of part of the food by an equivalent amount of dry matter from sprouted maize in the rations fed to bullocks brought about some improvement in the digestibility of the constituents of the rations.

Various investigators have shown that germination increases the amylase, protease, lipase, and other enzyme level several fold. Pett (412), University of Stockholm, observed that *germination markedly increases proteolytic activity* of wheat seeds and others claim it multiplies the amylase content of wheat and barley from 3 to 10 times. Consequently, it is safe to say that the improved digestibility brought about by addition of sprouted maize is due largely to ingestion of extra enzymes and not to any factor in vitamin B.

Some exact measurements on the effectiveness of various enzymes *in vivo* were recently made on the surgically prepared dog and on the normal human subject by the physiologist Ivy and associates, Northwestern University, and by the physiologist Selle, University of Texas. Quotation from Ivy, Schmidt, and Beazell (413): "In dogs with complete duodenal fistulae, with bile and pancreatic juice excluded, addition of malt amylase to a meal of cereal, appreciably facilitated gastric emptying because of the liquefying action of amylase. Addition of malt amylase increased digestion of the starch from a control value of 5 to 12 per cent to a value of 30 to 65 per cent (average increase 370 per cent). About 87 per cent of the amylase passed into the duodenum in active form in these experiments. When a diastatically equivalent amount of human saliva was substituted for malt amylase, it was shown that considerably more starch digestion resulted with malt amylase. This is due to the fact that ptyalin, which is inactivated at pH 4.5, does not act as long in the stomach as malt amylase, which is inactivated at pH 2.5. When the experiments were performed on dogs with incomplete duodenal fistulae and with pancreatic juice and bile excluded, which more closely simulated the normal in that there is more rapid rise in gastric acidity, 69 to 71 per cent of the malt enzyme was recovered from the duodenum in 30 minutes if given orally with water, whereas with milk 34 to 54 per cent of the enzyme was obtained. In experiments on human subjects performed so as to simulate a salivary deficiency (expectoration of saliva), addition of malt amylase to a cereal meal definitely augmented gastric digestion of starch in 7 out of 8 normal subjects. In human subjects, the amount of active amylase given with a cereal meal that passes into the intestine varied from 42 to 100 per cent (average 51 per cent). In human experiments in which salivary amylase was permitted to play its normal role, using a mixed meal, it was found that addition of malt amylase increased the gastric digestion of starch in four out of ten normal subjects. In the presence of a deficiency of pancreatic amylase and of an inadequate secretion of saliva, which might be due to defective ptyalin formation or to the boiling of food, addition of malt amylase to the meal is definitely indicated by our results."

In 6 dogs, *achylia pancreatica* was established by Beazell, Schmidt, and Ivy (414) by ligation of the pancreatic ducts. On a high starch diet, fecal starch varied from 18 to 39 per cent. Oral administration of malt amylase, fungus amylase, and pancreatin, markedly decreased the amount of fecal starch. *Malt amylase and fungus amylase* were about equally efficient, being distinctly *superior to pancreatin.*

Establishment of experimental *achylia pancreatica* by Schmidt, Beazell, Crittenden, and Ivy (415), using ligation of pancreatic ducts in 7 dogs, caused large fecal loss of nitrogen and fat which were decreased to the extent of 60 per cent and 59 per cent respectively by oral administration of pancreatin. Fecal bulk was reduced by 37 to 42 per cent.

In 10 totally depancreatized dogs, sustained by insulin and studied by Selle (416), administration of pancreatin with the food reduced the quantity of feces 30 to 60 per cent, increased the elimination time to approximately normal value, and reduced fecal nitrogen 30 to 60 per cent. Selle believes the presence of food in the stomach may offer protection to pancreatic enzymes from gastric juice, and, in this respect, the experiments *in vitro* differ fundamentally from these.

The *old experiments* performed *in vitro* to test the ability of enzymes to survive acid treatment, are *no longer considered applicable to physiological conditions within the organism.*

SUMMARY AND CONCLUSIONS

1—The primitive ancestors of man were *not* cooking animals. Before the era of cookery, physiological processes became integrated with a diet containing numerous materials including enzymes.

2—A growing body of evidence indicates that there is an intimate physiological relationship and interaction between enzymes, vitamins, and hormones in the organism, and that a subminimal intake is reflected in an altered balance and accompanying perverted activity.

3—*Enzymes*, like vitamins are *normal constituents* of all vegetable and animal tissue in the raw natural state. Hence it is obvious that all wild animals ingest enzymes with their food. The same was true of an early type of man before the age of fire and cookery. Consequently, in any question concerning the status of food enzymes in nutrition, the burden of proof rests on those choosing the position that food enzymes are superfluous. This untenable position postulates the inconsistency that food enzymes have left no imprint upon intricate physiological processes during countless eons of time in which the organism was bequeathed a full complement of food enzymes at every meal.

4—Unlike vitamins, *enzymes* are extremely *thermo-labile*, being completely destroyed by a few minutes of boiling. The official pasteurizing procedure of 1/2 hour of heating at 145 degrees F. kills all except a small portion.

5—Primitive cookery was not as thorough or efficient as modern procedures. Consequently enzyme destruction was less extensive in former times.

6—For a better explanation of certain problems of physiology, it is necessary to think of enzymes as biological entities possessed of corporeal and incorporeal fractions. All of the facts pertaining to enzymes cannot be accounted for if only a limited chemical view of their nature is entertained. The enzyme complex should be visualized as a material carrier charged with an energy factor.

7—Gut impermeability to enzymes *in vitro* has little resemblance to the mechanism of absorption of enzymes in the living intestine.

8—The following evidence is offered as proof that the *absorption of enzymes from the intestinal tract* into the organism is a *regular physiologic process.*

(a) The assumption that enzymes cannot be absorbed by the living intestine because the enzyme molecule is too large or complex to pass through the dead intestine is shown to be erroneous by these facts:
(1) *Yeast cells* including their contained enzymes are *absorbed.*
(2) *Bacteria with a full complement of enzymes are absorbed.*
(3) *Absorption of unsplit protein* occurs with pronounced *regularity.*

(b) Oral administration of large quantities of enzyme extracts causes excretion of large amounts of enzymes in the urine, but no significant variations in the blood serum enzyme level. *Evidence indicates that absorption occurs through the lymphatic system* and that if the storage facilities of the organism are momentarily overtaxed, the surplus is promptly excreted into the urine. Evidently the blood serum is not a proper medium for investigating this phenomena.

(c) Of the large quantity of enzymes poured into the gastrointestinal tract by the salivary glands, stomach, pancreas, and small intestine, only a small amount is recovered in the feces. It is possible to account for the remainder only on the assumption that the enzymes are reabsorbed.

(d) A successful defense of the theory that enzymes cannot be absorbed must embrace the illogical assumption that the organism can afford to waste by excretion with the feces the enormous quantities of enzymes poured every day, week after week, and month after month, into the gastrointestinal tract from the salivary glands, stomach, pancreas, and small intestine. As a matter of fact, the organism apparently cannot tolerate the loss of even the pancreatic secretion for more than a few weeks as is shown when the pancreatic juice and its enzyme contents are drained out of the body by means of an experimental pancreatic fistula, resulting in rapid emaciation and death. Death results also in human pancreatic fistula in a large proportion of cases. That *death is due to loss of enzymes* and not to a wastage of fluid and salts is suggested by the fact that no such fatal termination results from experimental or human biliary fistula, in cases where no enzymes are lost with the secretion. In biliary fistula, life can be maintained indefinitely with proper diet and care.

(e) *Oral administration of enzyme* extracts in human patients results in *improvement* in various systemic disturbances. There is no evidence that the reported benefits can be accounted for solely on the basis of improved digestion in the gastrointestinal tract. Considered together with the other evidence, it appears more likely that the ingested enzymes are absorbed into the body, there to exert their special effects, and that at least part of the therapeutic result is achieved directly in the tissues.

9—Normal human urine contains relatively more enzymes than normal blood serum. The urinary enzyme level is susceptible to wider physiologic variations in response to body conditions. Therefore, under controlled conditions, *urine* is a more sensitive and consequently *more satisfactory medium* in *investigations on the absorbability* of enzymes. The results of investigations utilizing blood serum in testing absorbability of enzymes must be evaluated with these facts in mind.

10—Since foods of high calorie values contain far more enzymes in the raw state than low calorie foods, it is *not possible to compensate for the enzymes lost in a heat-treated meal* of meat and potato, for instance, *by* an addition of raw vegetables such as a *salad*. This point requires special emphasis, because fruits and leafy vegetables are commonly utilized to balance the diet for vitamins and minerals.

11—While the enzyme value of a single meal of raw food is small, the sum total of enzymes in a raw food diet eaten during the course of a lifetime far exceeds not only the enzyme value of secreted digestive juices but also the enzyme value of the whole organism. It follows, that if exogenous enzymes are permitted to participate in the labors of digestion and metabolism less endogenous enzymes will be required.

Enzyme activity exacts a toll on the organism entailing daily loss of a certain amount of "spent" enzymes in the urine, feces, and sweat. *If no enzyme replacements* are taken in from the outside, the normal daily excretion of enzymes results in an *earlier depletion of the enzyme potential* of the body and consequently to earlier onset of senility and death.

12—Reported experimental evidence indicates that *enzymes are* secreted by the various glands in response to *specific* stimuli. Starchy foods stimulate amylase secretion, protein foods proteolytic enzymes, and fat foods cause more lipase to be secreted. This correlation with the nature of the food is confirmed by comparison of animal species in which the pancreas and the feces of carnivora contained more trypsin but less amylase than the pancreas and feces of herbivora. Further confirmation of this highly specific and adaptable reaction of the organism is supplied by the work of Abderhalden. It was shown, that when various materials are injected into the organism, distinctive enzymes appear in the urine which are highly specific for the type of material introduced. The particular relevance of this evidence upon the utility of food enzymes in the organism resides in the circumstance that if all of the ingredients of a meal are digested and reduced, before being eaten, to substances not requiring further digestion - if all carbohydrates are reduced to dextrose, proteins to peptones, and fats to fatty acids - then obviously there would be no work for the digestive enzymes of the body to do. Since the starch, protein, and fat which normally stimulate the secretion of digestive enzymes are absent, the enzyme potential is spared the necessity of supplying the corresponding enzymes full strength. Consequently the daily depreciation, as is evidenced by the appearance of "spent" enzymes in the urine, feces, and sweat, is lessened.

13—Determination of the degree of digestion of foodstuffs by the enzymes naturally present in the foods has been undertaken by various investigators. The digestive action of food enzymes was demonstrated both in the test tube and in the organs of living animals. *Food enzymes* were found to do a measurable amount of work and to that extent displace and *conserve* the *enzymes of the organism.*

14—Comparison of *enzymes* found in wheat, rice, barley, sugar cane, milk, honey, meat, and other *foods* with the same enzymes contained in the *digestive secretions* shows that they possess the *same* characteristics. The organism modifies the pH optimum according to its particular needs. Since the organism can transform vegetable protein into animal protein and vegetable starch into animal starch (glycogen), it is not too much to expect that plant and animal enzymes can likewise be absorbed and utilized since their modification is presumably a simpler problem.

15—The *incidence* of many *diseases* such as cancer, heart disease, diabetes, and arthritis continues upward in spite of increasing attention to the vitamin intake. While the realization that these diseases may have a nutritional background is gaining new advocates, it is important that all weapons in the armament be considered, including food enzymes. *Enzyme deficiency* is insidious enough to be suspected as a *causative factor*. Development of pernicious industrial practices has caused greater enzyme deficiency in the diet accompanied by a parallel increase in incidence of many chronic diseases.

16—The usual method of testing the vitamin value of food by animal feeding is insufficient to indicate the complete adequacy of a diet since the observations occupy only the early growing period of the life cycle, equivalent to the period of early maturity in human beings. The technique of vitamin essaying is faulty in so far as it fails to suggest the requirements for an optimum diet promoting long life and freedom from disease during the full period of the life span. The fact that a rat may display apparent good health during the virile growing period upon a supposedly adequate diet judged by vitamin standards is no proof that the same diet will be sufficient to maintain good health to an advanced age or even to middle life. On the contrary, feeding experiments extending throughout the life span of the animal have shown that *experimental animals develop many degenerative diseases in the later period of the life cycle when fed a diet supplemented only by vitamins.*

17—The fact that the pancreas of herbivorous animals, subsisting exclusively upon raw plant substances, is relatively very small (relatively less than half as large as the human) offers convincing testimony of the *important part played by food enzymes in digestion.* Not only is the pancreas small in herbivora, but in cattle and sheep the salivary glands are also inactive, furnishing no enzymes to assist in carbohydrate digestion whatsoever. And this inspite of the fact that the food of these herbivora is largely of a carbohydrate nature which would seem to indicate need for a large pancreas and highly active salivary glands. How is it possible to reconcile these various facts unless it is granted that the enzymes consumed with the food take over a large part of the digestion in herbivora?

18—Another link in the chain of evidence tracing effects to their causes is supplied by the illuminating behavior of the human and animal pancreas in response to extra work imposed by heat-treated, enzyme-deficient diet. The available evidence indicates that Orientals on a high carbohydrate cooked diet, essentially rice, display a pancreas approximately 50 per cent heavier than that of Americans. The salivary glands of Orientals are also larger. Organ weight studies on experimental animals show that when a group of rats (rats have active salivary glands) is placed upon a heat-treated, high carbohydrate diet and sacrificed after a period of feeding, the average weight of the pancreas and salivary glands shows a marked increase over a similar control group of animals on a mixed diet. This indicates that the pancreas and salivary glands are forced to undergo considerable hypertrophy to furnish the additional enzymes required, thus confirming experimentally in animals what has been observed in human beings. It is a singular circumstance that whereas cattle and sheep, ingesting a full quota of food enzymes, consummate the digestion of a comparatively high carbohydrate raw diet with only a small pancreas and without help from the salivary glands, human beings on a heat-treated mixed diet, lacking food enzymes, require a large pancreas and active salivary glands to digest a smaller amount of carbohydrate. And furthermore, a *high carbohydrate, heat-treated diet engenders still greater enlargement of the pancreas and salivary glands* in humans and animals.

19—Numerous reports disclose that increase in metabolic activity is paralleled by rise in the enzyme content of blood serum and increased enzyme loss in the urine. It is understandable, that if metabolism is essentially a function of enzyme activity, the organism mush forfeit some of its enzymes by loss through the urine, and the excretion of these "spent" enzymes is to be considered as a natural corollary of the price of such metabolic effort. This additional urinary *loss of enzymes* in instances of increased metabolism assumes special significance in evaluating the *shortened life span* of experimental organisms when exposed to elevated temperature, extra physical work, and increased food intake. The following conditions involving heightened metabolic activity display elevated blood serum enzyme values and increased elimination of enzymes in the urine:

Muscular work
Fevers
Increased food intake
Pregnancy

20—Observed sub-normality in enzyme content of body fluids is often cursorily relegated to failure of pancreatic function. In the light of the evidence unearthed, it appears not unlikely that the intrepid effort of the pancreas at compensation is sponsored by a fundamental default, i.e. failure of the food to supply the enzyme replacements necessary to prevent a strained hypertrophy of the pancreas.

21—It is interesting to note, that one of the main characteristics of enzymes is their accelerated activity with rising temperature, i.e. enzymes work faster at a fever temperature of 104 degrees F than at normal body temperature. There is much evidence to indicate that the *increased response of enzymes to elevation in temperature functions as the main mechanism of defense of the body against bacteria and other invading agents.* For, whereas bacterial activity decreases with increase in fever, enzyme activity increases with increase in fever. In this connection, it may be recalled that the white blood cell which protects against infection is endowed with a greater diversity of enzymes than any other cell. It is not unlikely that, mainly by virtue of its enzyme content, the white blood cell is enabled to display the digestive action against bacteria characteristic of phagocytosis.

22—Evidence is submitted indicating that a comprehensive test of the capacity of the animal organism to endure on an enzyme-free diet requires exclusion of exogenous enzymes gaining entrance through the agency of air borne bacteria, yeasts, and fungi. The efficiency of these unicellular organisms as enzyme producers has been widely demonstrated in industrial processes. There are good grounds for believing that the enzyme-deficient animal organism reluctantly offers a culturing abode to bacteria, yeasts, and fungi with the object of confiscating their enzymes. The evidence warrants a strong suspicion, that the unnatural *appropriativeness of enzyme-deficient organisms for exogenous enzymes* may invoke bacterial activity of intractable magnitude and *engender susceptibility to infections.* Due consideration should be accorded these factors in accounting for the widespread incidence of bacterial diseases.

23—A circumstance of no mean import is furnished by the studies of a number of investigators on the amylase content of the blood serum and urine of man and more than ten common species of animals. Human blood serum contained the smallest quantity of enzymes of any of the animals tested. And yet the amount of enzyme voided in human urine was comparable to the others, being out of proportion to the amount found in human blood serum. While it may be difficult to provide an exact interpretation of this interesting paradox, it is significant that an exceptionally low human blood serum content parallels a sizable loss of enzymes in the urine. There is an implication that the discrepancy is related to man's ingestion of a heat-treated, enzyme-deficient diet.

24—Even if one chose to ignore all evidence to the contrary, it would not be logical to assume that enzymes in food are non-essential. Indeed, it is impossible to prevent the enzymes existing in raw food from performing some of the labors of digestion which otherwise would be the burden of the enzymes of the digestive fluids. Enzymes in raw foods become active the very moment the cell walls are ruptured during the act of mastication and before the digestive enzymes have had time to function. Thus, any assumption that food enzymes are superfluous is contradictory.

25—The status of the pancreas and other enzyme-secreting glands requires clarification. The assumption is general that a few ounces of glandular tissue comprising the enzyme-secreting organs can supply the large quantities of enzymes elaborated every day. It is obvious that the pancreas cannot supply from its own substance the protein, salts, and water out of which pancreatic juice is made. Sober reflection suggests that the vital component of enzymes must likewise be supplied by food or by the cells of the organism and carried to the pancreas by the blood stream. Surgical grafts of gland tissue upon a host organism are speedily exhausted. The extensive migrations of white blood cells and their rich and diversified endowment of enzymes causes them to be logically looked upon as the main vehicles by which enzymes are conveyed to the pancreas or transported about in the organism. It is not inconceivable that white blood cells can transfer part of their enzyme energy from one protein to another by adsorption. The *pancreas is thus established as merely an assembling, conditioning, and disbursing organ.* Generally speaking, when the pancreatic juice is subnormal in enzyme content, it must not be interpreted merely as a local involvement of the pancreas, but as evidence of an enzyme deficiency condition in the cells of the whole organism.

26—Experimental pancreatectomy provides added proof of primary responsibility of the body tissues in maintaining optimum enzyme concentration in the blood serum and digestive secretions, and emphasizes the subordinate role played by the pancreas as an assembling, conditioning, and disbursing organ. The fall in the blood serum enzyme level consequent to pancreatectomy may be made to give way to a sudden rise to the preoperative level or even above it after injection of insulin. Such animals may live in a fair state of health for years without a pancreas, if suitable measures are employed. From whence come these enzymes that reestablish the proper blood serum level? It must be conceded that, under influence of endocrine guidance, the enzymes of the body are normally mobilized to be made use of according to current exigencies. Since there is a different optimal pH for enzymes in pancreatic secretion, blood serum, and body tissues, the powers of the organism in modifying enzyme characteristics are shown to be remarkable. There is *no justification*, therefore, based on this score, *for placing arbitrary limitations on the concept of absorption and utilization of food enzymes.*

27—Unless body tissues are recognized as the reservoir of digestive and blood enzymes, how is it possible to explain why the virgin tissues of an experimental animal can maintain a normal serum enzyme level with the pancreas completely removed, while the serum enzyme level of human beings with presumably devitalized tissues is frequently found to be lowered with the pancreas intact? If it be conceded that the pancreas and other secreting glands are dependent on body tissues for enzymes, especially for the vital fraction of the enzyme complex, then the capacity of the tissues in supplying this enzyme energy becomes a fertile field for investigation and assumes a high order of importance. This capacity, which may be designated as the *enzyme potential, is obviously fixed and limited*. To assume otherwise would deny natural law.

28—There are many points of identity between the enzyme potential and what is commonly known as vitality. The synonymy of this subtle power operating in the organism with the vital factor of the enzyme complex, enzyme energy, enzyme activity, metabolic activity, vital energy, nerve force resistance, life force, and what Professor Moore called "biotic energy" is rendered highly probable by the complexion of the evidence. With the exception of the enzyme concept all of these terms, including the commonly used "resistance", are vague and abstract, failing to denote a concrete or measurable entity. There is no justification, therefore, for continued use of such indefinite terminology. *Enzymes, being capable of exact measurement, emerge as the true yardstick of vitality*.

29—The life span of water fleas and fruit flies, kept at various temperatures, varied with the temperature. In a cold environment, not conducive to rapid exhaustion of enzymes and promoting sluggish physical activity, life lasted 108 days in water fleas, while at a temperature 20 degrees higher, where enzymes are used faster and where insects are very active, duration of life was only 26 days. At the warmer temperature, the life span was decreased about 400 per cent, but the heart beat was increased about 400 per cent. The *total number of heart beats* (some 15 million) in the life of a water flea is about the *same regardless of length of life*, showing that the organism has a fixed sum total of vitality or enzyme potential to spend.

30—The life span in fruit flies, water fleas, brook trout, and rats also varies according to the amount of food permitted. The amount of food necessarily determines the quantities of enzymes engaged. On a diet in which the quantity of food was not limited, entailing extra sacrifice of enzymes, the length of life was shortest. Where the amount of food was restricted to a quantity sufficient to prevent starvation, promoting *economical use of enzymes*, the *life span was markedly increased*, sometimes doubled.

31—The basal metabolism in fruit flies as well as in man has been found to decrease progressively with advancing old age.

32—There is evidence that longevity and maximum growth are incompatible. Rats and insects kept at reduced weights because of insufficient feeding lived longer.

33—Water fleas living on a diet limited in quantity, thus promoting a longer life span, had a slower heart rate than those maintained on a diet not limited in quantity and which engendered a shorter life. Independent confirmation of this experimental result has been achieved by Professor Pearl who divided 386 men, on whom records had been kept, into two groups according to the length of life. Each of the long-lived group averaged *26 years more* than the short-lived group. The *long-lived men had a heart rate 4 beats per minute less and a weight 6 pounds lower* on an average than the short-lived group. Extra enzymes are engaged and spent in promoting extra heart effort as well as by a surplus weight premium. This quickened drain on the enzyme potential to a level incompatible with the continuance of life causes a shorter life span.

34—Enzyme content of the whole macerated bodies of a long-living type of fruit fly was considerably greater than the enzyme content of a short-living type of fruit fly. The alleged influence of human ancestral strains upon longevity thereby finds some measure of confirmation, and the high rate of energy expenditure and unusual capacity for abuse of some persons with a history of ancestral longevity becomes explicable.

35—Enzyme content of the whole macerated bodies of flies and grass-hoppers is greatest at the period of early maturity and least in old age.

36—Enzyme content of the whole macerated bodies of beetles is also greatest in the young adult, decreasing to about half in the old beetle.

37—Enzyme content of the whole macerated bodies of rats is greatest at the adult stage, diminishing as age advances to a low point in old age.

38—The amylase content of human saliva was found to be 30 times greater on an average at 25 years of age than at 81 years of age.

39—The amylase content of human urine is considerably lower in old age than in younger persons.

40—Beetles maintained at an abnormally high temperature of 118 degrees F are very active at first and then gradually become dormant and appear to be dead. Tests on the whole bodies at hourly intervals showed gradual decrease of enzyme content. Enzymes working on a substrate *in vitro* behave similarly - higher temperatures induce increased performance but rapid destruction, lower temperatures decrease output but cause much slower destruction. Since the behavior of the animal organism under the influence of elevated temperature is identical with that of enzymes acting on a substrate in vitro, it can be *concluded that the life force and the enzyme potential are one and the same.*

41—The literature supplies evidence that there is no assurance that the increased rate of growth and height recorded in groups such as college students in recent years in relation to so-called improved nutrition is wholly favorable. Studies on school children have shown there is a tendency to incompatibility between maximum physical development and optimal health.

42—Comparison of the mineral composition of the tissues of old persons and of young persons dying of disease showed that, *in disease, changes similar to those occurring in old age tend to take place.*

43—Contrary to popular belief, the absolute length of life has not increased. Actually, fewer persons alive at 70 today survive until 90 than 40 years ago. This can be conveniently accounted for on the basis of decreased enzyme intake and increased rate of enzyme expenditure due to the augmented pace of living.

44—There are no recorded instances of well defined pathological lesions in wild jungle animals living in their natural habitat. Evidence as to the incidence of disease in wild animals held in captivity is abundant. In the past, when random indifferent feeding was the practice, the incidence of various diseases was high. Steep mortality rates took a sharp downward turn in zoo animals with the recent inauguration, particularly for valuable animals such as lions, tigers, and the anthropoids, of the raw food enzyme-containing diet, with spectacular improvement in reproduction, longevity, and decreased incidence of disease.

45—In a study of the weights of 17 organs of several hundred domesticated rabbits, it was found that there were decided changes in the weights of nearly all organs in rabbits presenting manifestations of disease of spontaneous origin. Disease, even in its mildest form, is capable of effecting the weights of organs that are not directly involved in the disease process, and the effect produced bears a relationship to both the extent and the activity of the lesions present.

46—Rat colonies maintained during their whole lives on conventional human-style diets, or even on diets supplemented artificially with minerals and vitamins, develop many pathological conditions not seen in rats during the abbreviated course of vitamin essaying. It is difficult to avoid the inference that the appearance of disease in long-term vitamin-supplemented diet experiments presages the need of the organism for all food constituents, including food enzymes, if optimal health and longevity are to be attained.

47—Differences in the health, physical condition, and life span between animals maintained on a heat-treated, vitamin-supplemented diet, and animals maintained on a raw, unheated diet can only be ascribed to extremely heat-labile factors of which enzymes are the chief representatives.

48—The activity displayed by enzymes in changing a substrate presumably involves the expenditure of energy. The theory, that enzymes act by their mere presence and are not used up in the process, has never been sufficiently explored. The evidence upon which it is based is not convincing. It would seem to be a denial of natural law.

49—Cooking tribes, such as the American Indian and jungle peoples, have a more or less comprehensive materia medica, the medicine man being a prominent member of the tribe. The contrast with the isolated *polar Eskimo* is striking since these inhabitants of the far north consume much of their food in the *raw uncooked* state and have *no* materia medica or *apparent need for a medicine man.*

50—With the knowledge now available on the significance of food enzymes, the attempt of Metchnikoff to explain the longevity of Bulgarian peasants by their domiciliation of a type of innocuous intestinal bacteria is seen not to have been well founded. A far better explanation is that a large part of the calorie intake of these long-lived people was in the form of raw foods richly endowed with enzymes. The dairy products consisting of sour milk, sweet milk, butter, and cheese which made up a large proportion of the diet were taken in the raw unpasteurized form. Therefore the drain on the enzyme potential was less than on the conventional heat-treated diet of the present day, and the peasants might have been expected to retain a *sufficiently high enzyme potential to maintain life to an advanced age.* Since the dairy foods are important sources of both calories and enzymes, the diet is seen to have been better balanced than the present diet of high-calorie, heat-treated foods and enzyme-poor fruits and vegetables.

51—Further light as to the significance of enzymes in food is provided by evidence obtained in a comparative study of the effects of raw human or cow's milk and pasteurized or otherwise heat-treated milk on babies and rats. In one study, comprising more than 20,000 babies in Chicago, 7 per cent of those dying were in the breast-fed group while 66 per cent were in the bottle-fed group. In another study in Boston, *mortality of breast-fed babies was only about 1/4 that of bottle-fed babies.* Raw milk conferred high immunity to dental caries in children. Bones of rats fed on raw milk had slightly higher content in calcium and phosphorus than the bones of rats fed on pasteurized milk, suggesting that the phosphatase content of raw milk and its absence in pasteurized milk may be an important factor. In second and third generation rats on pasteurized milk, there was loss of hair and the hemoglobin content of the blood was slightly less than in rats on raw milk. Several investigators direct attention to a growth-promoting factor in raw milk destroyed by pasteurization and not identifiable as any of the known vitamins. The fact that the pasteurizing temperature of 145 degrees F is highly destructive to enzymes but harmless to vitamins, except vitamin C, establishes the enzymes in milk as being the most likely antecedents of the superior effects reported for raw milk. Furthermore, vitamin C, which is reported not to be needed in the nutrition of the rat, is harmed only little, while enzymes are almost completely destroyed by pasteurization.

52—The primitive isolated Eskimo offers an excellent opportunity to test the validity of the food enzyme concept under conditions comparable to that of the controlled requirements of a laboratory experiment. The diet consists principally of meat, fish, and fowl. Most of the food is consumed *raw*, the remainder being eaten rare. Fish supplies a large share of the diet and is consumed raw after having been buried in pits during part of the winter and allowed to autolyze through the agency of its own enzymes, assuming characteristics not unlike some of our strong cheeses. The entire fish, including the enzymes contained in the digestive secretions, is eaten. The liver of seal is highly prized and is eaten raw as is the stomach contents of animals containing the digestive enzymes; also seal fat which contains a moderated quantity of lipase. The presence of lipase in seal fat helps explain why the Eskimo can metabolize fats so completely as to avoid ketosis, shown by absence of acetone in the urine. On an exclusive heat-treated protein and fat diet in civilized countries ketosis usually appears. *The health of the primitive Eskimo is excellent.* Evidence gathered from physical examinations, urinalysis, blood analysis, basal metabolism and roentgenological examination was almost 100 per cent negative in indicating any pathological condition. This is all the more remarkable when it is recalled that the meat consumption may reach 5 to 10 pounds daily. The living conditions also are such as are not customarily regarded as conducive to health. Conditions are strikingly different in the case of the *modernized Eskimo* who has been provided with a dry wooden house, given store clothing, and has opportunity to purchase modern foods at the store. Under these conditions *diseases are rife,* furnishing a remarkable contrast to the primitive Eskimo.

53—If an intelligible opinion is to prevail regarding the true nature of enzymes, it is essential to weigh not only an isolated portion of the evidence, but to assemble and coordinate all of the available chemical, medical, and biological facts whereby unrelated facts frequently supplement each other

54—The *therapeutic value* of various types of *raw diet* such as raw milk, raw fruit juice, raw vegetable juice, and raw fruit and vegetable has been established in many chronic and otherwise intractable diseases and reported by numerous physicians. There is a discernible undercurrent of opinion among practicing medical men, that a certain amount of raw uncooked food in the diet is indispensable to the highest degree of health. The special virtue of raw food is sometimes ascribed to its "live" quality - raw food being spoken of as live food. The evidence indicates that the unique value of the raw food diet resides in its enzyme content.

55—Excessive use of salt is generally regarded to be objectionable. It is demonstrable that various salts, including NaCl, stimulate enzyme activity in the test tube as well as in the digestive flow, and it is not inconceivable that the propensity of the organism for salt on a heat-treated diet is accentuated by a need for digestive enzymes. Cooked foods taste "flat" without addition of salt, and since digestive secretions do not flow properly in the absence of relish for food, it might be expected that digestion would be retarded. It has been shown, however, that on a raw food diet there is no need for table salt. Consequently, the excretion of chlorides in the urine is very low, but the blood chlorides are higher than on a heat-treated diet containing added salt, an unexpected and surprising finding! An added incongruity relates to the fact that *persons on salt-free raw diets have been shown to tolerate the sweating bath better than those on a heat-treated diet containing added salt.* In view of this disturbing evidence, it seems reasonable to reexamine the propriety of exclusive reliance on extra NaCl intake in occupations entailing exposure to heat and to advise use of more raw foods for such workers.

56—The *favorable influence of supplementary exogenous enzymes in diabetes* is duplicated by the mildly hypoglycemic action of raw food diets in the presence of hyperglycemia. That the effect is due to enzymes has been shown by the drop in sugar content following oral or intravenous administration of amylase or sucrase. Various raw substances containing enzymes such as yeast, liver, and egg yolk have been shown to decrease hyperglycemia and urinary sugar. So-called insuloids, which are heat-stabile, also exert marked hypoglycemic effects in diabetes. That the hypoglycemic action of enzymes is independent of insuloids is shown by the fact that ligation of pancreatic ducts in rabbits, dogs, and chickens, by increasing the serum-enzyme level, either lowered the blood sugar level or improved tolerance for carbohydrates. In view of the fact that the digestive secretions, blood, and urine in diabetes have frequently been reported low in enzyme content, the benefit following enzyme administration is not unexpected.

57—The singular results following use of supplementary exogenous enzymes in gastrointestinal, cardiovascular, and cutaneous diseases, in arthritis and sprue have been recited by the literature. Especially notable results have been attained in many conditions associated with a type of allergy allegedly caused by appearance in the blood stream of food materials not completely digested, according to the theory of the Oelgoetz school. In the presence of a high serum-enzyme level, the blood stream is supposed to act as a buffering medium to prevent the entrance of any adventitious matter into the tissues by completing its digestion. It has been established experimentally that *orally administered enzymes perform efficiently in the presence of deficient pancreatic or salivary digestion,* markedly decreasing the fecal loss of nitrogen, fat, and starch. Furthermore, it has been shown that orally administered enzymes can speed up digestion beyond the normal average.

CONDENSED SUMMARY AND CONCLUSIONS

1—*Enzymes are normal constituents of all cellular matter.*

2—Enzymes are far *more thermo-labile* than vitamins.

3—All wild animals live exclusively on raw food including a full quota of enzymes. So did an early type of man.

4—*Modern cookery destroys more enzymes* than in primitive times.

5—The enzyme complex is a biological entity composed of corporeal and incorporeal fractions. Enzymes and catalysts do not display all features in common.

6—Behavior of the dead intestine as regards permeability to enzymes is no criterion as to absorbability of enzymes by the living intestine.

7—Extensive *absorbability of enzymes is proved* by the following evidence:

(a) Yeast cells, bacteria, and unsplit proteins are absorbed.

(b) Orally administered enzymes are recovered in the urine.

(c) Large quantities of enzymes are secreted into the gastrointestinal tract, but only a small amount is recovered in the feces.

(d) Loss of pancreatic enzymes by experimental or human pancreatic fistula is rapidly fatal, invalidating the supposition that extensive fecal excretion of enzymes is tolerable. On the contrary, death is not inevitable in experimental or human biliary fistula where no enzymes are sacrificed.

(e) Oral administration of enzyme extracts to human patients results in improvement in systemic disease.

8--*Enzymes in raw foods take priority in digestion over secreted enzymes.* Exogenous or food enzymes become active the moment the cell wall is ruptured by mastication and before endogenous or secreted enzymes have made an appearance.

9—Endogenous enzymes are *secreted in response to specific stimuli* by starch, protein, fat, etc.

10—*Metabolism and digestion exact a toll* resulting in a depreciation of the enzyme potential and the excretion of "spent" enzymes in the urine, feces, and sweat.

11—If some digestion is performed by *exogenous enzymes,* the stimulus to secretion of endogenous enzymes is less intense. Consequently, there is *less drain on the enzyme potential.*

12—While the enzyme value of raw food is small, the sum total of enzymes available in a raw food diet consumed over a period of years far exceeds both the enzyme value of digestive secretions and the whole body.

13—Experimental evidence indicates that food enzymes do a measurable amount of digestive work in the test tube and in the organs of living animals.

14—The technique of vitamin essaying fails to ascertain that a diet which may be effective in maintaining health in the early life of the experimental animal will be equally effective in conserving health and preventing disease in the period of middle life and old age.

15—The pancreas of herbivorous animals is relatively only about one half as large as that of American adults and their salivary glands do not secrete enzymes, while human salivary glands are highly active. The fact that *herbivorous animals using enzyme-containing raw food can digest much carbohydrate food with only a small pancreas and no salivary enzymes,* while man, on a heat-treated enzyme deficient diet requires a large pancreas and active saliva, offers convincing testimony on the *utility of food enzymes.*

16—*The pancreas of Orientals on a heat-treated, high carbohydrate rice-type diet is relatively about 50 per cent heavier than that of Americans, and their salivary glands are also heavier.* This hypertrophy of the pancreas and salivary glands in response to higher intake of enzyme-deficient carbohydrate foods has been confirmed experimentally in animals.

17—Increase in metabolic activity such as muscular work, pregnancy, fever, and increased food intake is paralleled by rise in the enzyme content of blood serum and increased loss of "spent" enzymes in the urine.

18—Observed sub-normality in enzyme content of body fluids in disease cannot ultimately be relegated to failure of pancreatic function since it is traceable to a fundamental default, i.e. failure of a heat-treated diet to supply the enzymes necessary to maintain the enzyme potential of the tissues.

19—The *white blood cell is endowed with a greater diversity of enzymes* than other cells. The digestive action characteristic of phagocytosis is thereby better defined.

20—The *protective value* of fever is illustrated by the fact that bacterial activity decreases with increase in fever while *enzyme activity increases with increase in fever.*

21—Available evidence is interpreted as signifying that the animal organism can sequester and utilize the enzymes of bacteria when food enzymes are not available. The innocuousness of such behavior is open to serious doubt.

22—Of ten species of animals examined, human blood serum contained the smallest quantity of enzymes and yet the excretion of "spent" enzymes in human urine was about as great as in the animal urine. Considered together with the other evidence, there is an implication that the discrepancy is related to man's ingestion of a heat-treated enzyme-deficient diet.

23—Maintenance of a normal blood serum enzyme level after experimental pancreatectomy supported by insulin medication emphasizes the subordinate role played by the *pancreas and other enzyme-secreting organs as assembling, conditioning, and disbursing organs* only and points to the tissues as the ultimate reservoir of enzymes.

24—The synonymy of the subtle power operating in the organism with the vital factor of the enzyme complex, enzyme energy, enzyme activity, metabolic activity, vital energy, nerve force, resistance, and life force is rendered probable by the nature of the evidence. *Enzymes*, being capable of exact measurement, are the true yardstick of *vitality*.

25—That the *enzyme potential, vitality, and "resistance"* are one and the *same* entity is emphasized by the following evidence. The length of life is held to be inversely proportional to the rate of energy expenditure.

(a) Influence of temperature.

(1) Higher temperature increases the speed of enzyme reactions *in vitro* but brings about a correspondingly speedier inactivation of the enzyme.

(2) The higher temperature of fever causes extra loss of enzymes in the urine.

(3) Higher temperature increases the tempo of life in fruit flies and water fleas, measured by quickened movement, but also shortens the life span correspondingly.

(4) Evidence of approaching senility such as loss of hair, weight loss, decrease in length, wrinkling of the skin, sluggish movements, and failure in reproduction can be made to appear sooner or later in life depending on the rate of energy dissipation which is influenced by the temperature.

(5) Higher temperature increases frequency of the heart beat and CO_2 production in cold-blooded animals.

(6) Higher temperature increases the velocity of germination of seeds.

(7) Higher temperature increases the velocity of incubation of eggs.

(b) Influence of food.

(1) The amount of food consumption regulates the quantity of enzymes engaged and consequently determines the daily urinary toll. The amount of enzymes the organism must sacrifice daily through the

urine is influenced by the meals, there being a regular cycle of rise and fall with an immediate rise after a meal.

(2) Greater food consumption markedly decreases the life span in fruit fleas, water fleas, rats, and trout.

(3) Greater quantity or variety of food increases the height of college students and increases the weight of albino rats. More organic defects appear in school children with better physical development.

(c) Influence of heredity.

(1) A *long-living type of fruit fly has a considerably higher content of esterase and protease* than a short-living type.

(2) The hereditary influence in human longevity is generally recognized.

(d) Both enzyme content and viability in seeds diminish with age:

(e) Enzyme content of the whole macerated bodies of fruit flies, grasshoppers, beetles, and rats is greatest in early maturity, decreasing to a minimum in old age.

(f) *Enzyme content of human saliva and urine becomes markedly decreased in old age.*

(g) *Enzyme content* of body fluids is *diminished in many diseases.*

(h) Basal metabolism decreases in old age.

(i) There is incompatibility between maximum growth and physical development on the one hand, and maximum length of life, good health, and freedom from physical defects on the other.

(j) Changes in the chemical composition of the tissues in disease are similar to the changes occurring in old age.

26—Jungle animals are free from degenerative disease. The formerly high mortality and morbidity in zoo animals has taken a steep downward turn with the advent of the raw food diet.

27—Changes in weight of organs occasioned by disease are accompanied by compensatory weight alterations of all the organs and the development of related symptomatic phenomena.

28—The appearance of *disease* in long-term, vitamin-supplemented diet experiments utilizing *heat-treated food* presages the need of the organism for all food constituents, including food enzymes.

29—Differences in the health, physical condition, and life span between animals maintained on a heat-treated, vitamin-supplemented diet, and animals maintained on a raw, unheated diet can only be ascribed to extremely heat-labile factors of which enzymes are the outstanding representatives.

30—There is a striking contrast between cooking tribes, such as the primitive American Indian, requiring a comprehensive materia medica and the *raw-diet consuming Eskimo with no medicines* or apparent need for them.

31—The legendary longevity of Bulgarian peasants, ascribed by Metchnikoff to innocuous intestinal bacteria, can be more satisfactorily explained on the basis of the enzymes contained in the predominantly raw diet of dairy products.

32—Discrepancies between breast-fed and bottle-fed babies in mortality and morbidity, and incidence of caries and the differences in hemoglobin content and bone content of calcium and phosphorus of rats fed on raw or pasteurized milk can be considerably ascribed to the moderate quantities of several *enzymes contained in raw milk* but which are almost completely *lacking in pasteurized milk.*

33—*The high health standards of the primitive isolated Eskimo contrasted with the soaring morbidity of the modernized Eskimo offers an unparalleled example of the utility of enzymes in food supply.* The diet of the primitive Eskimo contains large quantities of whole fish including all of the enzymes of gastric juice, pancreatic juice, and intestinal juice; liver, and stomach contents of animals including gastric juice and its enzymes; and great amounts of raw meat. The remarkable absence of ketosis on a diet high in protein and fat and low in carbohydrate is probably related to the ingestion of enzymes with the food including lipase in seal fat.

34—The *therapeutic* efficacy of several types of *raw food* diet has been established and its unique value is found to reside in its *enzyme* content.

35—Universal craving for salt on a heat-treated diet is thought to be accentuated by the necessity for increased enzyme activity which is stimulated by salt. A possible obnoxious influence of salt ingestion is indicated by the fact that on a raw food saltless diet the urinary elimination of chlorides is very low while the blood chlorides remain exceptionally high.

36—The hypoglycemic or hypoglycosuric action of enzymes has been demonstrated by oral or intravenous administration of enzyme preparations, by consumption of enzyme-containing raw foods, and by increasing the serum-enzyme level through experimental pancreatic or salivary duct ligation.

37—Successful enzyme therapy of a number of ailments has been reported. *Orally administered, enzymes perform efficiently in the digestive tract and display considerable digestive activity* even in the presence of a normal concentration of endogenous enzymes.

GLOSSARY of SCIENTIFIC TERMS

Achylia: absence of Hydrochloric acid and pepsin in gastric juice.

Acidosis: pathological condition in the body due to accumulation of acid or loss of base.

Adipose: of a fatty nature.

Adrenal: situated near the kidney.

Adventitious: found at unusual place.

Afebrile: without fever.

Albumin: a specific water soluble protein in nearly all animals and many plants.

Albuminuria: presence of serum albumin in urine.

Albumose: albumin containing carbohydrate.

Amylase: enzyme that catalyze hydrolysis of starch into smaller molecules.

Amylolytic: pertaining to promotion of digestion or disintegration of starch.

Amylopsin: a-amylase of pancreas.

Angina pectoris: spasmodic, choking or suffocative pain.

Anorexia: lack or loss of appetite.

Apical: pertaining to or located at the apex.

Arteriosclerosis: diseases due to thickening and loss of elasticity of arterial walls.

Asepsis: freedom from infection; prevention of contact with microorganisms.

Aseptic: sterile.

Atoxic: not poisonous.

Atrophy: a wasting away, diminution in size.

Autoclave: an apparatus for sterilization under pressure by steam.

Autolysis: spontaneous disintegration of cells by own enzymes.

Avitaminosis: a condition due to deficiency of one or more vitamins.

Biliary: pertaining to bile, bile duct or gall bladder.

Ca: calcium.

Cachectic: general ill health and malnutrition condition, see Cachexia.

Cachexia: pronounced state of constitutional disorder.

Carapace: hard outer covering as the upper shell of a turtle.

Carbohydrate: compounds of carbon, hydrogen & oxygen; e.g., starch, cellulose, sugars.

Casein: a phosphoprotein, the principal milk protein and basis of curd and cheese.

Catabolism: any destructive process by which complex substances are converted by living cells into simpler compounds.

Catalase: an enzyme catalyzing decomposition of hydrogen peroxide of cells.

Catarrhal: pertaining to inflammation of a mucous membrane, especially of head and throat.

Cathepsin: a protease found in most cells; splits peptide bonds; also active in self digestion of tissues.

Caudal: general term to refer to a tail like structure or appendage.

Cerebellum: back part of brain concerned with coordination of movements.

Cerebrum: main portion of brain constituting the largest part of nervous system.

Cholecystitis: inflammation of the gall bladder.

Cholinesterase: an enzyme catalyzing the conversion of acetylcholine to choline.

Chyle: consists of lymph and droplets of triglyceride fat in a stable emulsion, absorbed through intestine from food, gets mixed with blood.

Cirrhosis: a chronic liver disease.

Cisterna chyli: a dilated portion of thoracic duct at its origin in the lumbar region.

Cl: Chloride.

CO_2: carbon dioxide.

Coagulation: clot formation; formation of a gelatinous mass.

Colitis: amebic dysentery.

Colloid: glutinous or gelatinous suspension in liquid.

Colostrum: thin, yellow, milky secretion of mammary gland few days before or after birth.

Controls: a standard against which experimental observations are made varying only one factor.

Cu: copper.

Dehydration: removal of water from a substance.

Dehydrogenase: an enzyme facilitating transfer of hydrogen in biochemical reactions.

Dermatitis: inflammation of the skin.

Dermatoses: skin diseases, especially ones without inflammation.

Dextrose: obtained by hydrolysis of starch, white powder with sweetish taste.

Diastase: enzyme responsible for conversion of starch into maltose and then into dextrose.

Dipeptidase: an enzyme hydrolyzing the peptide bond of a dipeptide.

Duodenitis: inflammation of the duodenum.

Duodenum first or proximal portion of small intestine.

Dysfermatosis: a skin affliction.

Dysmenorrhea: painful menstruation.

Dyspepsia: impairment of the power or function of digestion.

Dystrophy: any disorder arising from defective or faulty nutrition, especially muscular dystrophies.

Eck fistula: artificial passage made between portal vein and vena cava.

Eczema: superficial inflammation with redness, itching, weeping, oozing, crusting, scaling.

Edema: presence of excessive fluid between cells, especially in the subcutaneous tissues.

Endocrine gland: any ductless gland, e.g. thyroid, adrenal, whose secretions pass into blood directly.

Entelechy: a supposed vital principle as a directive spirit.

Enteritis: inflammation of the intestinal tract.

Eosinophilic: readily stainable with Eosin, a rose colored dye.

Erepsin: a group of enzymes hydrolyzing partially digested proteins in small intestines to amino acids.

Erysipelas: contagious skin disease caused by *Streptococcus pyogene.*

Erythrocytes: red blood cells or corpuscles.

Esterase: enzyme catalyzing hydrolysis of ester to acid and alcohol.

Euglobulin: a class of proteins insoluble in water but soluble in saline solution.

Exanthematous: pertaining to any eruptive disease or eruptive fever.

Fe: iron.

Febrile: pertaining to fever.

Fibrin globulin: insoluble protein predominantly forming blood clot.

Fistula: an abnormal duct or passage from an abscess, cavity , or a hollow organ.

Gastric anacidity: achlorhydria, lack of normal gastric acidity.

Gastric Atony: lack of normal tone or strength of the stomach.

Gastric mucosa: mucous membrane of the stomach.

Gastric Neuroses: disorder of gastric digestion due to nervous system disturbance.

Gastritis: inflammation of the stomach.

Globulin: any of a class of water insoluble proteins found in milk, blood, muscle, plant seeds, etc.

Glucagon: a pancreatic polypeptide hormone involved in blood sugar regulation.

Glycerol: a sugar alcohol, pharmaceutical preparation called glycerin.

Glycogen: chief animal storage carbohydrate primarily in the liver.

Glycosuria: abnormal excretion of glucose in urine.

Gram: 1/28 of an ounce.

Grave's disease: disorder of thyroid mostly in women.

H2S: hydrogen sulfide, a chemical reagent.

HCl: hydrochloric acid.

Hematopoiesis: formation and development of blood cells.

Hemoglobin: the oxygen-bearing, iron containing protein in vertebrate red blood cells.

Hydration: the process or condition of combining with water.

Hydrogen ion: hydrogen atom without electron. The more hydrogen ions in a solution, the more acid that solution is.

Hyperthermia: abnormally high body temperature.

Hypertrophy: enlargement of organ due to increase in size of constituent cells.

Hypoglycemia: abnormally diminished content of glucose in the blood.

Hypothermia: abnormally low body temperature.

Hypovitaminosis: condition due to deficiency of one or more vitamins.

in vitro: within a glass, in an artificial laboratory environment.

in vivo: within living organism.

Instar: any stage of an anthropod between shedding of an outer covering and development of a new one.

Insulin: pancreatic hormone that regulates carbohydrate metabolism by controlling blood glucose levels.

Insuloids: compounds having insulin like activity.

Invertase: an enzyme acting on a specific kind of carbohydrate .

Jejunal: pertaining to small intestine between duodenum and ileum.

K: potassium.

KCN: potassium cyanide, an extremely poisonous substance.

Kidney: responsible for filtering blood and excreting waste through urine; regulates sodium, potassium, phosphate and other ions in extracellular fluid.

Lactase: enzyme hydrolyzing lactose sugar of milk.

Lacteals: any of the intestinal lymphatics that transport chyle.

Lactose: milk sugar.

Lesion: any traumatic discontinuity of tissue or loss of function of a part.

Leukemia: disease characterized by distorted proliferation of leuko-cytes and precursors in blood and bone marrow.

Leukocytes: White blood cells which are also responsible for fighting disease in the body.

Leukocytosis: increase in number of white blood cells resulting from disease.

Ligation: application of a ligature to tie a vessel or strangulate a part.

Ligature: any substance such as catgut, cotton, silk or wire used to tie a vessel or strangulate a part.

Lipase: enzyme catalyzing hydrolysis of ester linkage of fats.

Lipoid: fat like.

Lipolytic: pertaining to splitting up of fat molecules.

Lipoma: a benign tumor usually composed of fat cells.

Liver: filters and stores blood, converts sugars into glycogen and stores it, secretes bile, etc.

Lung infarcts: area of coagulation death of tissue due to impeded circulation in lung.

Lymph: transparent slightly yellow alkaline liquid derived from tissue fluids, found in lymphatic vessels.

Macerated: softened by wetting or soaking.

Maltase: an enzyme responsible for hydrolyzing glucose sugar to glucose.

Metabolism: sum of physical and chemical processes by which living organized substance is produced and maintained, and also the transformation by which energy is made available for the usage of the organism.

Methylbutyrase: an enzyeme which acts on methylbutyl groups.

Mg: magnesium.

Mikulicz's disease: a benign, self limited lymphocytic infiltration and enlargement of the lachrymal and salivary glands.

Milligram: 1/1,000 of a gram. An ounce is 28 grams.

Mitosis: method of indirect division of a cell; process of growth and replacement of cells.

mL: 1/1,000 of a liter. A pint is 473 mL.

Mn: manganese.

Morbidity: diseased; or the ratio of sick to healthy persons in a community.

Myocardial: pertaining to muscle tissue of heart.

N: Nitrogen.

Na: sodium.

NaCl: chemical symbol for common table salt.

Nasopharyngeal: pertaining to that part of larynx which lies above the level of soft palate.

Nephritis: any of various acute or chronic inflammations of kidney.

Neuralgic: paroxysmal pain along the course of one or more nerves.

Nuclease: enzyme involved in splitting nucleus into simpler constituents.

^{o}C: Degrees Celsius. On this scale water boils at 100°, and freezes at 0°.

^{o}F: Degrees Fahrenheit. On this scale water boils at 212°, and freezes at 32°.

Oxidase: enzyme that catalyzes reduction of molecular oxygen independently of hydrogen peroxide.

P: phosphorus.

P-poisoned: phosphorus poisoned.

Pancreas: secretes digestive enzymes, secretions insulin and glucagon regulate blood carbohydrates.

Pancreatectomy: surgical removal of the pancreas.

Pancreatin: substance obtained from pancreas of hog or ox, contains amylase, protease, lipase enzymes.

Papain: a protease enzyme from latex of papaya.

Paraplasm: abnormal growth.

Parenterally: not through digestive tract, but other routes, like subcutaneous, intravenous, etc.

Paresis: slight or incomplete paralysis.

Parotid gland: a gland situated near the ear.

Pathological: structural and functional changes of tissue and organs by disease.

Pecilothermic: ability to change and adapt body temperature to environment.

Pepsin: catalyzes split of peptide bonds in proteins.

Peptidase: category of enzymes hydrolyzing peptide linkages.

Peptide: chemically bonded amino acids, e.g., a dipeptide contains two amino acids, tripeptide has three, etc. Proteins consist of hundreds, or thousands of amino acids.

Peptide Bond: the chemical bond formed between two amino acid moieties by removal of one molecule of water.

Peptolytic: splitting up of peptones which are obtained from partial digestion of proteins.

Pericarditis: inflammation of pericardium, the fibrous sac surrounding the heart.

Peristalsis: worm-like propelling of contents inside tubular organs, like digestive tract.

Pernicious anemia: decrease in number of red blood cells in persons with manifestation of malabsorption of vitamin B12 due to failure of gastric mucosa to secrete adequate and potent intrinsic factor.

Peroxidase: enzymes which catalyze oxidation in presence of hydrogen peroxide.

pH: measure of acidity/alkalinity. pH 7 is neutral. 7—>0 acidity increases. 7—>14 alkalinity increases.

Phagocytosis: engulfing of microorganisms, other cells and foreign particles by phagocytes, such as leukocytes.

Phlorodnized: glycosuria caused by usage of phloridzin from root bark in experimental animals.

Phosphatase: enzyme hydrolyzes mono-phosphoric esters to inorganic molecules.

Pituitary: governing endocrine gland.

Plasma: fluid portion of blood in which particulate components are suspended.

Plasmolysis: shrinking of protoplasm in cell due to loss of water by osmotic action.

Polymorphonuclear: having a nucleus deeply lobed or so divided that it appears to be multiple.

Presbyopia: impairment of vision due to old age, near point of distinct vision moves farther away from the eye.

Protease: general term for enzymes cleaving peptide bonds in proteins or peptides.

Proteins: complex combinations of literally hundreds or thousands of alpha amino acids; principal constituents of cell protoplasm.

Proteolytic: splitting of peptide bond between amino-acids in proteins to give smaller molecules called polypeptides.

Pruritus: itching; also conditions characterized by itching.

Pseudoglobulin: class of globulin proteins soluble in water.

Psoriasis: chronic, hereditary, recurrent disease of scalp, elbows, knees and shins.

Ptyalin: a-amylase enzyme in saliva.

Puerperal: pertaining to period or state of confinement after labor.

Saccharase: an enzyme acting on a specific kind of carbohydrate .

Scleroderma verum: chronic hardening and shrinking of connective tissue.

Senescence: condition resulting from the transitions and accumulations of the deleterious aging processes.

Serum Albumin: a major protein of human blood plasma.

Spleen: acts in formation and as a reservoir of red blood cells. Also other undetermined important functions.

Sprue: chronic form of malabsorption syndrome.

Starch: complex carbohydrate from various plant tissues.

Subcutaneous: beneath the skin.

Submaxillary: beneath the bone of the lower jaw.

Substrate: a substance on which an enzyme acts.

Substratum: a lower layer.

Succus entericus: the liquid secreted by the glands in the wall of small intestine.

Sucrase: an enzyme acting on sugar.

Sucrose: common sugar.

Suprarenal: situated above kidney.

Systolic: pertaining to contraction of heart, especially ventricles.

Thiry-vella: artificial opening into an internal closed loop of intestine, which communicates with abdominal wall through an intestinal segment interposed between surface and loop.

Thoracic: pertaining to or affecting the chest.

Toxicosis: disease condition due to poisoning.

Tributyrinase: enzyme cleaving tributyrin.

Trypsin: a specific protease from pancreas.

Urease: enzyme causing change of urea to carbon dioxide and ammonia.

Urticaria: vascular reaction of skin marked with elevated patches and severe itching.

Vegetative neurosis: acrodynia; a disease of infancy and early childhood.

Vena cava: main trunk of vein near heart.

Vena portae: portal vein, a short thick trunk connecting with pancreas and liver.

Vestigial: of the nature of a vestige, trace or relic; rudimentary.

Villi: small vascular protusions from free surface of a membrane.

Visceral: pertaining to any large interior organ in abdomen, thoracic region etc.

Viscometric: pertaining to viscosity of a substance.

REFERENCES

1. McCay et al, J.*Nutrition*, 10:63-79(1935)
2. Stefansson, J.*Amer.Dietet.Assoc.*, 13:102-19(1937)
3. Westenbrink, *Arch. neerland. Physiol.*, 20:116-22(1935)
4. Shuger and Arnold, *Proc. Soc.Exp.Biol.Med.*, 29:494-6(1931-32)
5. Fisher, *Proc. Soc.Exp.Biol.Med.*, 28:948-51(1930-31)
6. Fisher, *Proc. Soc.Exp.Biol.Med.*, 29:490-94(1932)
7. Tychowski, *compt.rend.soc.biol.*, 104:538-40(1930)
8. Alexander et al, J.*Clin.Invest.*, 15:163-67(1936)
9. Ratner, *Amer.J.Physiol.*, 109:86-7(1934)
10. Ratner & Gruehl, J.*Clin.Invest.*, 13:517-32(1934)
11. Wilson & Walzer, *Amer.J.Dis.Children*, 50:49-54(1935)
12. Crandall, *Amer.J.Digest.Dis.&Nut.*, 2:230-5(1935)
13. Oelgoetz et al, *Amer.J.Digest.Dis.&Nut.*, 3:159-61(1936)
14. Oelgoetz et al, *Medical Record*, Oct. 21, 1936
15. Oelgoetz et al, *Amer.J.Digest.Dis.&Nut.*, September 1934
16. Oelgoetz et al, *Amer.J.Digest.Dis.&Nut.*, December 1934
17. Virtanen & Soumalainen, *Zeit.Physiol.Chem.*, 219:1-21(1933)
18. Boldyreff, *Quart.J.Exp.Physiol.*, 10:115-201(1916)
19. Sansum, *Southwestern Medicine*, 16:452-62(1932)
20. Renda, *Semena Medica*, 2:1190-3(1924)
21. Elson, *Urol. & Cutan.Review*, 39:408-10(1935)
22. Sellei, *Urol. & Cutan.Review*, 41:112-5(1937)
23. Sellei, *Klin.Woch.*, 13:1725-27(1934)
24. Masumizu, Tohoku J.*Exp.Med.*, 5:1-11(1924)
25. Kallo, *Zeit.ges.exp.Med.*, 86:848-53(1933)
26. Kallo, *Frankfurt. Zeit.Pathol.*, 48:305-9(1935)
27. Kokuryo, *Japan J.Med.Sci.*, 2:115-30(1933)
28. Cohen, *Brit.J.Exp.Pathol.*, 6:173-9(1925)
29. Cameron, *Med.J.Australia*, 1:91-4(1923)
31. Reid, *Brit.J.Exp.Pathol.*, 6:314-26(1925)
32. Carlson & Luckhardt, *Amer.J.Physiol.*, 23:148-64(1908)
33. Wohlgemuth, *Biochem.Zeit.*, 21:81-422(1909)
34. Kleinmann & Sharr, *Biochem.Zeit.*, 251:275-328(1932)
35. Schlesinger, *Deut.Med.Woch.*, 34:593-5(1908)
36. Moeckel & Rost, *Zeit.Physiol.Chem.*, 67:433-85(1910)

37. Myers & Reid, *J.Biol.Chem.*, 99:595-605(1933)
38. Watanabe, *Amer.J.Physiol.*, Vol. 45, Dec. 1917
39. Boldyreff, *Skand.Arch.Physiol.*, 49:96(1926)
40. Ivanov & Basilewitsch, *Zeit.ges.exp.Med.*, 55:107-10(1927)
41. Wohlgemuth, *Grundriss der Fermentmethoden*, Berlin J.Springer Verlag, 1913
42. Howell, *Text-Book of Physiology*, 7th Ed.
43. Villaret & Justin-Besancon, *Nutrition*, 6:209-22(1936)
44. Sampogna, *Zent.Biochem.Biophys.*, 13:609
45. Harrison & Lawrence, *Brit.Med.J.*, 1:317-9(1923)
46. Morabito, *Pediatria Revista*, 37:1335-42(1929)
47. Gerner, *Hospitalstid*, 74:963-74(1931)
48. Gray & Samogyi, *Proc.Soc.Exp.Biol.Med.*, 36:253-5(1937)
49. Zucker et al, *Amer.J.Physiol.*, 102:209-21(1932)
50. Engelhardt & Gertschuk, *Biochem.Zeit.*, 167:43-53(1926)
51. Neilson & Lewis, *J.Biol.Chem.*, 4:501-6
52. Nielson & Terry, *Amer.J.Physiol.*, 15:406 (1906)
53. Samytschkina, *Pflugers Arch.*, 230:680-8(1932)
54. Simon, *J.Physiol.et Pathol.gen.*, 9:261 (1907)
55. Evans, *Biochem.Zeit.*, 48:442-7(1913)
56. Piccaluga, *Studium*, 21:427-32(1931)
57. Goldstein, *Arch.Verdauungskrankh*, 40:56-75(1927)
58. Koldayev, *Charcov.Med.J.*, 1:37(1916)
59. Romijn, *Acta Drov.Neerland.Physiol.Phar.,Micro.*, 3:93-4(1933)
60. Krzywanek & Schakir, *Biochem.Zeit.*, 220:342-7(1930)
61. Abramson, *Acta Med.Scand.*, 86:478-85(1935)
62. Abderhalden, *Fermentforschung*, 12:129-79(1932)
63. Abderhalden, *Fermentforschung*, 12:229-43(1932)
64. Abderhalden, *Fermentforschung*, 13:291-7(1932)
65. Abderhalden, *Fermentforschung*, 13:505-43(1932)
66. Abderhalden, *Fermentforschung*, 13:544-62(1933)
67. Abderhalden, *Fermentforschung*, 14:43-53(1933)
68. Abderhalden, *Fermentforschung*, 14:76-104(1933)
69. Abderhalden, *Fermentforschung*, 14:443-61(1935)
70. Abderhalden, *Fermentforschung*, 15:49-93(1936)
71. Abderhalden, *Fermentforschung*, 15:93-120(1936)
72. Molinar, *Deut.Med.Woch.*, 43:326-9(1917)
73. Andreev & Georgiewsky, *J.Biol.Med.Exper.U.S.S.R.*, 14:51-8(1930)

74. Andreev & Georgiewsky, *Arch.ges.Physiol. (Pflugers)*, 230:33-41(1932)
75. Andreev & Georgiewsky, *Arch.ges.Physiol. (Pflugers)*, 235: 428-37(1935)
76. Mangold & Dubiski, *Arch.Tierer Tierz.*, 4:507-25(1931)
77. Schwarz & Teller, *Fermentforschung*, 7:229-46(1924)
78. Aron, *Biochem.Zeit.*, 9:163-84(1908)
79. Grimmer, *Biochem.Zeit.*, 4:80-98(1907)
80. Boas, *Klin.Woch.*, 9:2295-6(1930)
81. Matveev, *Therap.Arch.,U.S.S.R.*, 12:140-4(1934)
82. Reichert, *The Differentiation and Specificity of Starches*, published by The Carnegie Institution, Washington, DC
83. Mangold, *Biochem.Zeit.*, 156:3-4(1925)
84. Pozerski, *Bull.soc.sci.hyg.aliment.*, 21:1-29(1933)
85. Roseboom & Patton, *J.Vet.Med.Association*, 74:768(1929)
86. Roseboom & Patton, *Amer.J.Physiol.*, 100:178(1932)
87. Buddle, *Zeit.Kinder.*, 46:195-209(1928)
88. *Anat. Record*, 32:119-32(1926)
89. *Yearly Average Weights, Chicago Stock Yards*
90. Private Communication by Dr. Fenger, Armour & Co.
91. S.Sisson, *Textbook of Veterinary Anatomy*
92. *Philosophical transactions Crisp*, 1865
93. Sitsen, *Mededeel Dienst Volksgezondheid Nederlandsch-Ind.*, 3:490-9(1927)
94. Sitsen, *Anthropologischer Anzeiger*, 7:103(1931)
95. DeLeon et al, *Philippine J.Sci.*, 52:97-127(1933)
96. Jackson, *Morris Human Anatomy*, 8th Ed., 1925.
97. Schaefer, *Anatomical Record*, 32:119-32(1926)
98. John, *J.Amer.Med.Assoc.*, 101:184-7(1933)
99. Flaum, *Klin.Woch.*, 11:1704-5(1932)
100. Flaum, *Wien.Arch.inn.Med.*, 23:201-22(1932)
101. Glaser & Bannet, *Klin.Woch.*, 12:345(1933)
102. Jackson, *J.Nutrition*, 3:61-77(1930)
103. Brown, Pearce & Van Allen, *J.Exp.Med.*, 42:163-78(1925)
104. Brown, Pearce & Van Allen, *J.Exp.Med.*, 43:241-62(1926)
105. Brown, Pearce & Van Allen, *J.Exp.Med.*, 44:85(1926)
106. Dehlhougne, *Deut.Arch.Klin.Med.*, 165:213-22(1929)
107. Gerner, *Bibliotek for Laeger*, 123:437-70(1931)

108. Kreyberg, *Norsk.Mag.Laegevidenskap*, 5:992-1003(1926)
109. Pavel et al, *Wiener Arch.innere Med.*, 28:133-44(1935)
110. Thomsen, *Ugeskrift for Laeger*, 91:1045(1929)
111. Pfeiffer, *Zeit.ges.exp.Med.*, 47:386-405(1925)
112. Solovtzova, *Russky Vrach*, 16:569-601(1917)
113. Spinelli, *Minerva med.*, 1:201-7(1932)
114. Frohlich & Neumann, *Wien.Arch.inn.Med.*, 27:245-62(1935)
115. Eckhardt, *Jahrb. fur Kinderheilk*, 142:319-43(1934)
116. Eckhardt, *Deut.Arch.Klin.Med.*, 177:517-26(1935)
117. Bach & Lustig, *Magyar Orvosi Archivum*, 32:301-13(1931)
118. Ma, *Monat.Kinder.*, 36:363-76(1928)
119. Bohmig, *Wien.Arch.inn.Med.*, 14:129-48(1927)
120. Solaroli, *Arch.fisiol.*, 37:69-96(1937)
121. *Amer.J.Physiol.*, 56:408-14(1921)
122. Burge, *Amer.J.Botany*, 15:412-5(1928)
123. Viale, *Rend.accad.Lincei.*, 33:314-5(1924)
124. Burge & Neill, *Amer.J.Physiol.*, 47:13-24(1918); (124a)55:301-2(1921);
     55:299-301(1921); 61:574-76 (1922); 63:545-7(1923)
125. Pett, *Biochem.J.*, 29:1898-1904(1935)
126. Wasteneys, *Biochem.J.*, 30:1171-82(1936)
127. Swanson, *Cereal Chemistry*, 12:89-107(1935)
128. Jono, *Acta Scholae Med.Univ.Imp.Kioto*, 13:211-38(1931)
129. Vercesi, *Folia gynaecol.*, 18:309-29(1923)
130. Katsu, *Japan J.Obst.Gyn.*, 16:2-8(1933)
131. Ammon & Schutte, *Biochem.Zeit.*, 275:216-33(1935)
132. Koebner, *Zeit.ges.exp.Med.*, 76:792-803(1931)
133. Hileman & Courtney, *J.Dairy Sci.*, 18:247-57(1935)
134. *Biochem.Zeit.*, 166:172-89(1925)
135. *Arch.wiss.prakt.Tier.*, 58:375-84(1928)
136. *Proc.Soc.Exp.Biol.Med.*, 32:564-6(1934)
137. Kendall, *Boston Med. & Surg.J.*, 163:322(1910); Wisconsin Med.J.,
     June 1913
138. Levin, *Skandinavisches Arch.Physiol.*, 16:249(1904)
139. Corson-White, *Disease in Captive Wild Animals and Birds*,
     J.B.Lippincott & Co., 1923
140. Reid & Meyers, *J.Biol.Chem.*, 99:607-13(1933)
141. Schlesinger, *Deut.Med.Woch.*, 34:593-5(1908)
142. Moeckel & Rost, *Zeit.Physiol.Chem.*, 67:433-85(1910)

143. King, *Amer.J.Physiol.*, 35:301-32(1914)
144. LoMonaco, *Boll.soc.ital.biol.sper.*, 2:215-8(1927)
145. Wohlgemuth, *Biochem.Zeit.*, 21:391-431(1909)
147. Northrop, *Physiol.Rev.*, 17:144-51(1937)
148. Willstatter, *Chem.Rev.*, 13:501-12(1933)
149. Compton, *Proc.Roy.Soc.London*, 87:245(1914)
150. *Biochem.J.*, 7:26-622(1913)
151. *Biochem.Zeit.*, 219:30-50(1930)
152. *J.Am.Chem.Soc.*, 41:231(1919)
153. *J.Gen.Physiol.*, 2:215(1920)
154. *J.Biol.Chem.*, 38:229(1919)
155. *J.Inst.Brewing*, 39:487-93(1933)
156. *J.Indian Inst.Sci.*, 13:159-64(1930)
157. *J.Indian Inst.Sci.*, 14:47-50(1931)
158. *J.Indian Inst.Sci.*, 12:185-90(1929)
159. *J.Indian Chem.Soc.*, 11:339-50(1934)
160. *Mem.Coll.Agr.Kyoto Imp.Univ.*, 6:23-53(1928)
161. *Ind. & Eng.Chem.*, 23:71-4(1931)
162. *Zeit.Unter.Leben.*, 71:311-8(1936)
166. *Biochem.Zeit.*, 21:131(1909)
167. *Zeit.Exp.Path.Therap.*, 8:398(1910)
168. *Biochem.Zeit.*, 57:84(1913)
169. *Zeit.Physiol.Chem.*, 197:42-54(1931)
170. *Biochem.Zeit.*, 241:316-63(1931)
171. *Biochem.Zeit.*, 251:275-328(1932)
172. *Naturwissenschaften*, 17:85(1929)
173. *Invest.Tzen.Nauch-Issle.inst.Koz.Prom.*, 24: No. 2, 1932
174. *Biochem.Zeit.*, 81:109(1917)
175. *Fermentforschung*, 1:533(1916)
176. *J.Biol.Chem.*, 31:201(1917)
177. *Biochem.J.*, 10:130(1916)
178. *Biochem.J.*, 30:549-57(1936)
179. *Klin.Woch.*, 7:163-5(1928)
180. *Zeit.ges.exp.Med.*, 69:179-92(1929)
181. *Biochem.Zeit.*, 212:53-9(1929)
182. *Zeit.ges.exp.Med.*, 76:792-803(1931)
183. *Biochem.Zeit.*, 64:13(1914)
184. *Biochem.Zeit.*, 193:18-38(1928)

185. *Nagoya J.Med.Sci.*, 3:51-73(1928)
186. *J.Biol.Chem.*, 105:199-219(1934)
187. *J.Biol.Chem.*, 108:421-30(1935)
188. *J.Am.Chem.Soc.*, 55:320-4(1933)
189. *Zeit.Physiol.Chem.*, 146:151-7(1925)
190. *J.Agr.Chem.Soc.Japan*, 11:68-76(1935)
191. *Biochem.Zeit.*, 36:280(1911)
192. *Zeit.Physiol.Chem.*, 204:259-82(1932)
193. *Zeit.Physiol.Chem.*, 186:212-22(1930)
194. Moore, *Biochemistry-A Study of the Origin, Reactions and Equilibria of Living Matter*, Longmans,Green & Co. 1921
195. Troland, *Cleveland Med.J.*, 15:377(1916)
196. Ekman, *Ann.Soc.Zool.Bot.Fennicao Vanamo*, 10:1-141(1930)
197. Laird, *Medical Record*, 101:535-40(1922)
198. Willstatter, *Chem.Rev.*, 13:501-12(1933)
198. Wohlgemuth, *Biochem.Zeit.*, 21:432-46(1909)
199. Waldschmidt-Leitz & Reichel, *Zeit.Physiol.Chem.*, 204:197(1931-32)
200. Giri, *Biochem.Zeit.*, 275:106-11(1934)
201. Sherman, Caldwell & Adams, *J.Biol.Chem.*, 88:295-304(1930)
202. S.Morgulis, *Fasting and Under Nutrition*, E.P.Dutton & Co., New York, 1923
203. Willstatter & Rohdewald, *Zeit.Physiol.Chem.*, 221:13-32(1933)
204. Willstatter & Rohdewald, *Zeit.Physiol.Chem.*, 185:267-80(1929)
205. Kleinmann & Scharr, *Biochem.Zeit.*, 251:275-328(1932)
206. Stern, *Zeit.Physiol.Chem.*, 204:259-82(1932)
207. Iglauer, *Folia Hematol.*, 44:159-68(1931)
208. Konn, *Tohuku J.Exp.Med.*, 17:31-8(1931)
209. Motai, *Nagoya J.Med.Sci.*, 3:51-73(1928)
210. Kleinmann & Rona, *Biochem.Zeit.*, 241:283-363(1931)
211. Willstatter & Bamann, *Zeit.Physiol.Chem.*, 180:127-43(1929)
212. Willstatter et al, *Zeit.Physiol.Chem.*, 186:85-96(1929)
213. Hamburg & Pickholz, *Brau-Malzind*, 34:75-101(1934)
214. Chrzaszcz et al, *Biochem.Zeit.*, 160:155-71(1925)
215. *Cereal Chem.*, 11:551-6(1934)
216. *Zeit.Physiol.Chem.*, 204:89-100(1932)
217. *Biochem.J.*, 30:342-4(1936)
218. Tychowski & Polak, Biochem.Zeit., 192:463-78(1928)
219. Reyniers, Personal communication

220. Wohlgemuth, *Biochem.Zeit.*, 9:10-43(1908)
221. Hirata, *Biochem.Zeit.*, 47:167-83(1913)
222. Mayer, *Bull.Johns Hopkins Hospital*, 64:246-7(1929)
223. Gernhardt, *Zeit.Klin.Med.*, 124:153-67(1933)
224. Emerson & Helmar, *J.Lab.Clin.Med.*, 19:504-6(1934)
225. Meyer et al, *Amer.J.Physiol.*, 119:600-2(1937)
226. Saigusa, *Naval Med.Assoc.Bull.Tokyo*, Vol. 1, Oct. 1919
227. Harrison & Lawrence, *Lancet*, 204:169-70(1923)
228. Kreyberg, *Norsk.Mag.Laegevidenskap*, 5:992-1003(1926)
229. Morabito, *Pediatria Rivista*, 37:1335-42(1929)
230. Gerner, *Hospitalstid*, 74:963-74(1931)
231. Gray & Somogyi, *Proc.Soc.Exp.Biol.Med.*, 36:253-5(1937)
232. Dehlhougne, *Deut.Arch.Klin.Med.*, 165:213-22(1929)
233. Tomioka, *J.Gastroenterology*, 3:1093(1928-29)
234. Elman, Arneson & Graham, *Arch.Surg.*, 19:943-67(1929)
235. Wakefield & McCaughan, *Arch.Int.Med.*, 45:473-78(1930)
236. Voit & Pragal, *Munch.med.Woch.*, 82:1031-2(1935)
237. Polland & Bloomfield, *J.Clin.Invest.*, 9:107-13(1930)
238. Dehlhougne, *Klin.Woch.*, 5:2457-9(1926)
239. Bettolo, *Rass.terap.patol.olin.*, 4:No.6, 1933
240. Ryu, *J.Chosen Med.Association*, 24:305-13(1934)
241. Sugiyama, *Sei-i-kai Med.J.*, 54:1531-8(1935)
242. Balo & Lovas, *Virchow's Arch.path.Anet.klin.Med.*, 288:326(1933)
243. Green, *Biochem.J.*, 28:16(1934)
244. Lombardo & Anselmo, *Ann.Clin.Med.e.Med.Sperim.*, 19:373-80(1929)
245. Okada et al, *Proc.Imp.Acad.Tokyo*, 4:134-5(1928)
246. Van Steenis, *Nederland.Tij v Geneesk*, 78:1529-36(1934)
247. Sanguigno, *Rinascenza Medica*, 13:16(1935)
248. Volodin, *Arch.Verdauungskrankh*, 49:168-200(1931)
249. Barbera & Adinolfi, *Policlinico*, 43:27-41(1936)
250. Harrison & Lawrence, *Brit.Med.J.*, 1:317-19(1923)
251. Cameron, *J.Metabolic Res.*, 3:754-7(1923)
252. Paganelli, *La chin.med.Ital.*, 49:141-50
253. Bassler, *Amer.J.Dig.Dis. & Nut.*, Vol. 1 (1934-5)
254. Schmerel, *Biochem.Zeit.*, 208:415-27(1929)
255. Fearon, Dublin J.Med.Sci., 562:149-83(1918)
256. Wynhausen, *Derl.Klin.Woch.*, 46:1406(1909); 47:2107(1910)

257. Brinck & Gulzow, *Zeit.Klin.Med.*, 131:747-58(1937)
258. Lewis & Mason, *J.Biol.Chem.*, 44:455(1920)
259. Reid & Narayana, *Quart.J.Exp.Physiol.*, 20:305(1930)
260. Cohen, *Amer.J.Physiol.*, 69:125(1924)
261. Reid, Quigley & Myers, *J.Biol.Chem.*, 99:615-23(1933)
262. Markowitz & Hough, *Amer.J.Physiol.*, 75:571(1925)
263. Ottenstein, *Biochem.Zeit.*, 240:328-56(1931)
264. Gray & Somogyi, *Proc.Soc.Exp.Biol.Med.*, 36:253-5(1937)
265. Pernice, *Zeit.Kinderheilk*, 58:86-94(1936)
266. Rachmilewitz, *Amer.J.Dig.Dis.*, 5:184-9(1938)
267. Kuznetzov & Michailova, *Arch.Verdauungskrankh*, 40:41-55(1927)
268. Berger et al, *Klin.Woch.*, 14:490-6(1935)
269. Garry, *Arch.klin.Chirug.*, 174:378-96(1933)
270. Schemensky & Geling, *Arch.Verdauungskrankh*, 52:427-34(1932)
271. Probstein, Gray & Wheeler, *Proc.Soc.Exp.Biol.Med.*, 37:613-15(1938)
272. Koehler, *Calif. and Western Med.*, 48:247-51(1938)
273. Ivy, *Amer.J.Dig.Dis. & Nut.*, 3:677-81(1936)
274. Markowitz & Hough, *Amer.J.Physiol.*, *75:571*(1926) ??? see #220
275. Milla, *Boll.soc.ital.biol.sper.*, 9:835-7(1934)
276. Gayda, *Arch.Sci.biol.*, 90:165-70(1934)
277. Johnson & Wies, *J.Exp.Med.*, 55:505-9(1932)
278. Zuckor et al, *Amer.J.Physiol.*, 102:200-21(1932)
279. Fiessinger et al, *Enzymologia*, 1:145-50(1936)
280. Fiessinger et al, *Compt.rend.soc.biol.*, 112:549-50(1933)
281. Tsudzimura, *Arch.ges.Physiol.(Pflugers)*, 234:250-4(1934)
282. Diena, *Internat.Beitr.Ernahr*, 5:405(1919)
283. Pearl, *The Rate of Living*, A.A.Knopf, New York, 1928
284. Pearl, *Amer.Natur.*, 63:37-67(1929)
285. Colp, *Ann.Surg.*, 78:725-44(1923)
286. Berg & Zucker, *Proc.Soc.Exp.Biol.Med.*, 29:68-70(1931)
287. Laqua, *Bruns.Beitr.Klin.Chir.*, 150:507-16(1930)
288. McCaughan, *Amer.J.Physiol.*, 97:459-66(1931)
289. Herrin, *J.Biol.Chem.*, 108:547-62(1935)
290. Walters, Kilgore & Bollman, *J.Amer.Med.Assoc.*, 86:186-91(1926)
291. Bottin, *Rev.belge.sci.med.*, 7:394-434(1935)
292. Hawkins & Whipple, *J.Exp.Med.*, 62:599-620(1935)
293. Thanhauser et al, *J.Biol.Chem.*, 121:715-19(1937)
294. Heymann, *J.Exp.Med.*, 64:471-83(1936)

295. Pepper, *J.Econ.Entomol.*, 27:290(1934)
296. Loeb & Northrop, *J.Biol.Chem.*, 32:103-21(1917)
297. Terao & Tanaka, *J.Imp.Fisheries Inst.Tokyo*, 25:67(1930)
298. MacArthur & Baillie, *J.Exp.Zool.*, 53:221-42(1929)
299. Barett, *US Dept.Agriculture, Technical Bulletin* 553
300. Pearl, *Quart.Rev.Biol.*, 3:391-407(1928)
301. Gowen, *J.Gen.Physiol.*, 14:463-72(1931)
302. Bodine, *J.Exptl.Zool.*, 34:143-48(1921)
303. MacArthur & Baillie, *J.Exp.Zool.*, 53:243-68(1929)
304. Albergo, *Minerva Med.*, 23:678-82(1932)
305. McCay, *Anat.Record*, 57:102(1933)
306. McLester, *Canad.Med.Assoc.J.*, 33:6-10(1935)
307. *The Rat. Memoirs of the Wistar Institute of Anatomy and Biology*, Philadelphia, 1924
308. Northrop, *J.Biol.Chem.*, 32:123-6(1917)
309. McCay et al, *J.Nutrition*, 1:233-46(1929)
310. Ingle et al, *J.Exptl.Zool.*, 76:325-52(1937)
311. Burge & Burge, *J.Exptl.Zool.*, 32:203-6(1921)
312. Bodine, *J.Exptl.Zool.*, 34:143-8(1921)
313. Sekla, *Brit.J.Exp.Biol.*, 6:161-6(1928)
314. Falk, Noyes & Sugiura, *J.Gen.Physiol.*, 8:75(1925)
315. Mayer, *Bull.Johns Hopkins Hospital*, 44:246-7(1929)
316. Finizio, *Rev.Hyg. et Med.Infant.*, 8:224-9
317. Meyer et al, *Amer.J.Physiol.*, 119:600-2(1937)
318. Loeschke, *Jahrb.Kinderheilk.*, 146:133-75(1936)
319. Pernice, *Zeit.Kinderheilk*, 58:86-94(1936)
320. McClure & Chancellor, *Zeit.Kinder*heilk, 11:483-96
321. Dhar, *J.Physiol.Chem.*, 30:378-82(1926)
322. Dhar, *Quart.Rev.Biol.*, 7:68-76(1932)
323. Gafafer, *Pub.Health Rep.US Treas.Dept.*, 51:831-41(1936)
324. Simms & Stolman, *Science*, 86:269-70(1937)
325. Bernstein, *Cold Spring Harbor Symposia*, 2:209-17(1934)
326. Orr et al, *J.Hygiene*, 35:476-97(1935)
327. Jespersen et al, *Res.Lab.Vet.Agric.Coll.Copenhagen*, 166th Rep. pp106(1936)
328. Thompson & Hargrave, *J.Minist.Agric.Engl.*, 42:1123-7(1936)
329. Kohlman, Eddy, White & Sanborn, *J.Nutrition*, 14:9-19(1937)
330. McCollum, *Amer.J.Pub.Health*, 24:956-8(1934)

331. *Milk Plant Monthly*, June 1938
332. Grulee, Sanford & Herron, *J.Amer.Med.Assoc.*, 103:735-9(1934)
333. Glazier, *New England J.Med.*, 203:626
334. Ederton, *Ann.Eugenics*, 5:326-36(1933)
335. Sprawsen, *Agric.Progress*, 10:139-48(1933)
336. Catel, *Deut.Med.Woch.*, 61:985-8(1935)
337. Catel, *Wien.med.Woch.*, 86:1299-1300(1936)
338. Lasby & Palmer, *J.Dairy Sci.*, 18:181-92(1935)
339. Channon & Channon, *J.Hygiene*,
340. Potter, *Milk Diet as a Remedy for Chronic Disease*
341. Mattick & Golding, *Lancet*, 231:702-6(1936)
342. Elvehjem, Hart, Jackson & Weckel, *J.Dairy Sci.*, 17:763-70(1934)
343. Okada & Sano, Japanese *J.Exp.Med.*, 12:169-98(1934)
344. Arthus, *Arch.internat.Physiol.*, 43:131-53(1936)
345. Richet & Richard, *Bull.Inst.Oceanographique*, 478:3(1926)
346. Morgan & Kern, J.*Nutrition*, 7:367-79(1934)
347. Thomas, *J.Amer.Med.Assoc.*, 88:1559(1927)
348. Heinbecker, *J.Biol.Chem.*, 80:461-75(1928)
349. Shaffer, *J.Biol.Chem.*, 47:449(1921)
350. Nephriakhin & Berezin, *Repts.Astrakhan Volgo-Caspian-Sea Sci.Sta*, 7:88-99(1931)
351. Garber, *Hygeia*, 16:242(1938)
352. Price, *Dental Cosmos*, 77:841-6(1935)
353. Urquhart, *Canad.Med.Assoc.J.*, 33:193-6(1935)
354. Rabinowitch, *Canad.Med.Assoc.J.*, 34:487-501(1936)
355. Rabinowitch & Smith, J.*Nutrition*, 12:337-56(1936)
356. King, Kugelmass & Boedecker, *J.Amer.Dental Assoc.*, 21:110-25(1934)
357. Loewy & Behrens, *Klin.Woch.*, 9:390-2(1930)
358. Glassner, Wiener *Klin.Woch.*, 49:144-7(1936)
359. Eimer, *Klin.Woch.*, 11:203-6(1932)
360. *Jahrbuch fur Kinder*, 134:368-9(1932)
361. Just, *Deut.Med.Woch.*, 62:1086-9(1936)
362. Bircher-Benner, *Zeit.Ernahrung*, 2:130-8; 169-76(1932)
363. Bircher-Benner, *The Prevention of Disease by Correct Feeding.*, Food Education Soc., London 1933
364. Hackh, *Pacific Dent.Gaz.*, 38:817(1930)
365. Copiscarow, *Chemistry & Industry*, 53:534-5(1934)

366. Copiscarow, *Chemistry & Industry*, 56:566-7(1937)
367. Protti, *Boll.soc.ital.biol.sper.*, 8:1412-17(1933)
368. *Vet.J.*, 90:368-74(1934)
369. Leven & Butin, Questions of *Nutrition* U.S.S.R., 3:100-4(1934)
370. Sherman, *Scientific Monthly*, 43:97-107(1936)
371. Dove, *American Naturalist*, 69:469-544(1935)
372. Eimer & Kaufmann, *Deut.Arch.Klin.Med.*, 173:314(1932)
373. Stohr, *Zeit.ges.exptl.Med.*, 95:55-66(1934)
374. Eimer & Voigt, *Zeit.Klin.Med.*, 112:477-527(1930)
375. Rosenthal & Ziegler, *Arch.Int.Med.*, 44:344-50(1929)
376. Bufano, *Arch.farmacol.sper.*, 44:22-32(1927)
377. Holland et al, *Zeit.ges.exp.Med.*, 93:62-8(1934)
378. Cohen, *Amer.J.Physiol.*, 69:125-31(1924)
379. Rosefeld, *Klin.Woch.*, 10:637-9(1931)
380. Rosefeld, *Klin.Woch.*, 12:711(1933)
381. Geness & Epstein, *Arch.exp.Path.Pharmak.*, 171:733-43(1933)
382. Jones, *Medical Record*, 49:720-4(1896)
383. Reid & Narayana, *Quart.J.Exp.Physiol.*, 20:305-11(1930)
384. Deichmann-Grubler & Myers, *Biochem.Zeit.*, 288:149-54(1936)
385. Wilson & Strieck, *Biochem.Zeit.*, 251:199-203(1932)
386. Ottenstein, *Klin.Woch.*, 10:1114-6(1931)
387. Halprin, *New Jersey Med.J.*, 31:28-9(1934)
388. Vannocci, *Sperimentale*, 82:335-41(1928)
389. Bassler, *Med.Times and Long Island Med.J.*, 33:115-20(1933)
390. Milliken, *Texas State J.Med.*, 29:307-10(1933)
391. Wolffe, *Med.J.& Rec.*, 138:243-44(1933)
392. Walker, *Canad.Med.Assoc.J.*, 29:396(1933)
393. Brown, *Amer.J.Med.Sci.*, 161:501(1921)
394. Fiessinger & Gajdos, *Arvosi Hetilap*, 80:314-16(1936)
395. Schweitzer, *Urol.Cutan.Rev.*, 335(1936)
396. Bodechtel & Kinkin, *Munch.med.Woch.*, 82:413-16(1935)
397. Mostel, *Wien. med.Woch.*, 86:474-5(1936)
398. Palombi, *Terapia*, 24:353-8(1934)
399. Dell'Acqua, *Zeit.ges.exp.Med.*, 71:245-50(1930)
400. Nephriakhin & Berezin, *Repts.Astrakhan Volgo Caspian Sea Sci.Station*, 7:88-99(1931)
401. Belkina & Kremlev, *Z.exptl.biol.Med.*, 8:329-41(1928)
402. Messerli, *Schweiz.Zeit.Hyg.*, 12:789-91(1932)

403. Minz & Schilf, *Zeit.Ernahrung*, 2:311-14(1932)
404. Maignon, *Compt.rend.soc.biol.*, 86:1172-5(1922)
405. Maignon, *Bull.Acad.vet.France*, 5:283-8(1932)
406. Maignon, *Presse Med.*, 42:313-5(1934)
407. Maignon, *8 ieme.Reunion de l'Assoc.des Physiologistes, Nancy*, May 1934
408. Maignon, *Cong.internat.de l'Union therap.*, 1:390-8(1937)
409. Turkeltaub et al, *Problems of Nutrition*, Moscow, 5:121-34(1936)
410. Hervey, *Science*, 62-247(1925)
411. McCandish & Struthers, *Scottish J.Agriculture*, 21:141-6(1938)
412. Pett, *Biochem.J.*, 29:1898-1904(1935)
413. Ivy, Scmidt & Beazell, *J. Nutrition*, 12:59-83(1936)
414. Beazell, Schmidt & Ivy, *J. Nutrition*, 13:29-37(1937)
415. Schmidt, Beazell, Crittenden & Ivy, *J. Nutrition*, 14:513-30(1937)
416. Selle, *J. Nutrition*, 13:15-28 (1937)

Appendix I

AN INTERVIEW WITH THE AUTHOR

(First published in the 1980 edition)
Questions formulated and posed by
Viktoras Kulvinskas, M.S.,
Raw Food Nutritionist, Author and Lecturer

Did you find a receptive audience 40 years ago when your book first came out? What was the attitude of the medical profession at that time?

I believe most people coming into contact with the book and not studying it in detail, believed it was some sort of catalog for the National Enzyme Company, which published it. Many ordinary medical practitioners had no interest in the subject or did not feel qualified to comment on it. But those who took it upon themselves to speak for the profession, sometimes irresponsibly claimed, as they do now, that the digestive secretions are richly endowed with enzymes, and therefore can digest all food without aid from outside enzymes. This is, of course, only too true, but in contrast, it is also the precise kind of teaching that prevents the conquest of cancer and allows intractable disease free reign. This kind of advice assumes that enzymes have nothing more important to do than digest food, forgetting all of their numerous jobs in running the metabolism. It ignores completely THE LAW OF THE ADAPTIVE SECRETION OF ENZYMES which has been recently established and confirmed in scores of university laboratories. In the book ENZYME NUTRITION the subject of enzyme secretion is thoroughly covered. I have brought in overwhelming scientific evidence proving that the oversight, causing some of the spokesmen who take it upon themselves to speak for science in the careless language of the unscientific and discredited past, is doing the very thing that will keep chronic disease in the saddle indefinitely and force cancer drives for funds to be a perpetual and never-ending enterprise. Those studying the book ENZYME NUTRITION must come to the conclusion that anyone who preaches that our inside enzymes are all we need, and belittles outside enzymes must be blamed for encouraging killer diseases to take millions of lives, and intractable diseases keeping their deadly and painful grip over the lives of many more millions.

Continuing with the question, I have not heard from many people about the book so I am not in a very good position to state what the reaction was. There were only two thousand books published. About fifty went on the shelves of universities in this country and abroad. The book was indexed in Chemical Abstracts and Biological Abstracts, the bibles of scientific periodical literature. In one letter, Dr. Sergius Morgulis, Professor of Biochemistry, University of Nebraska College of Medicine, wanted some references to the scientific literature mentioned in the book. He said that many years ago he was attending a scientific convention in Copenhagen and the subject of food enzymes was the topic of discussion. He could not remember the name of the author or the title of the scientific report.

Over the years I inadvertently ran across some mention of speculation that the enzymes in food may have some effect on digesting it in the body. These words may sound encouraging but unfortunately they did not help to solve related physiological problems. One day early in my studies I was checking the periodical literature in Index Medicus for reports on the influenza epidemic during the first world war. In two reports published in a British medical journal, a doctor blamed a lack of food enzymes in the diet for influenza. I coined the term food enzymes, but this doctor *used* it fully fifteen years before. At that time, Index Medicus did not have a proper subject index, so I had to discover this report purely by accident. I have recently had some correspondence with Dr. Alsoph H. Corwin who manifested an intense interest in supplemental enzymes. I understand he is now retired but that he was professor of chemistry at an eastern university, perhaps Cornell. Tony Collier or Conner can check this. I have corresponded with many doctors over the years. National Enzyme Company has these records. I do not think you will get many opinions from medical doctors about food enzymes because they do not like to say anything about a subject they do not understand.

All of the correspondence relating to the book was received by the National Enzyme Company because they are the publishers. There is one outstanding personality that should be mentioned. In one of the indexing and abstracting publications I learned that food enzymes were discussed in a Symposium at the Second Joint Meeting of the German Nutrition Society, The Austrian Society for Nutritional Studies, and The Swiss Society for Nutritional Studies, held at Constance, September 1968. One of the reports was issued by Professor R. Ammon, M.D., Ph.D., Director of the Institute of Physiological Chemistry, University of Homburg/Saar, and entitled, "*Have Food Enzymes An Importance In Nutrition?*" The Report was published in a Supplement to the *Journal of Nutritional Sciences* (*Zeitschrift für Ernahrungswissenschaft* 8:1-142 (1969). I have a photocopy of the report.

In it the Professor is in full agreement that food enzymes have a part to play in digestion and metabolism. This is in sharp contrast to the opinions sometimes carelessly sputtered out by uninformed but influential people in this country. More than forty years ago I wrote and got a copyright on a little treatise called *ENZYMOLOGY* which was later reprinted and widely distributed by National Enzyme Company. The records would show how many copies of this informative booklet were given away - I would guess 50,000. If you do not have a copy, you should get one. If you place *ENZYMOLOGY* and the professor's report side by side you will be amazed at the similarity.

There can be little question that *ENZYMOLOGY* alerted the world to *ENZYME NUTRITION*. It is obvious that Dr. Ammon must have gotten his hands on a copy and supplemented its material with a great deal of his own data in making up the report. *ENZYMOLOGY* did not bear my name as the author, so there was no one to credit as the source of the information, which is the customary procedure in scientific reports. That food enzymes were given careful scientific scrutiny is shown when Dr. Ammon reported he found that plant enzymes are superior when taken orally. That they escaped damage in the stomach and intestine was proven when he recovered some of them in the feces. Other reports in the Symposium showed that the scientists tested plant enzymes in the stomach and found more of them passed through unharmed.

A couple of months ago I received a phone call from a research man in Loma Linda University in California. He was engaged in research to develop the ideal human diet and chose to use the gorilla as a model because this primate has a gastrointestinal tract somewhat similar to the human. He made several phone calls for information on anatomical, physiological and nutritional data and I finally gave him enough information to serve as a basis for his work project.

A few weeks ago a man from a college in Texas telephoned and said he already had a lower college degree, but must write a thesis for a master of arts degree in nutrition. He chose the subject intestinal autointoxication and needed as many references to the scientific literature as possible. I had made exhaustive searches of the scientific periodical literature on many aspects of *ENZYME NUTRITION*, but intestinal autointoxication was not one of them. Library research in this area is much like looking for a needle in a haystack. When he called back I gave him a number of references that were on file and he thanked me profusely. As you mentioned in your Introduction, the world is slowly getting around. These people must go to a great deal of trouble finding my phone number. I don't know how they get it.

What are some of the directions of research and new projects in which you are presently involved?

I would like to discuss some of these projects in detail for a sufficient audience. Some of them are discussed in a preamble for the formation of THE AMERICAN FOOD ENZYME CONCEPT RESEARCH FOUNDATION, INC., of which Mr. Charles E. Conner is organizer. He can furnish details.

Do you feel raw food diets are not only useful therapeutically but also can be an excellent maintenance diet, or do you feel that for most folks some cooked food is desirable?

Some animals such as bees and ants are very active and constructive, but the larger animals do only sufficient work to keep alive. We may say that only humans work for prolonged periods at a sustained pace, which might be considered unnatural. This extra work output requires more food. Authorities such as Professor Pearl taught that sustained hard physical work, especially in later life, shortened the life span. It is not difficult to supply the carbohydrate portion of the food needed with raw food. But raw fat and protein in palatable, usable forms are rather hard to get for the busy worker. When an individual does hard work all day, rest is expected and there is little enthusiasm to spend much time preparing food. The protein and fat needs are most conveniently met by use of cooked animal products such as meat and eggs, at the cost of their enzymes. The well known drawback to the usage of meat by humans is its putrefaction in the intestine. The relative length of the gastrointestinal tract compared to the length of the subject from the occiput to the coccyx is about 3 in carnivora, about 11 in primates and man, and 30 in herbivora such as cattle. It has been argued that food such as meat, which putrefies rapidly, is innocuous in carnivora because it is promptly excreted by the short intestine of carnivora, but remains in the longer human intestine long enough to become a possible health hazard.

Protein and fat can also be supplied by raw tree nuts and other seeds and in superior quality. But these have enzyme inhibitors which must be neutralized, usually by germination. Almost everyone can eat a few raw, ungerminated nuts without feeling discomfort from the inhibitors. But if tree nuts are to be used in sufficient quantity to displace other proteins and fats, the enzyme inhibitors must be neutralized. Experiments on growing young rats and chicks have shown that heavy intake of enzyme inhibitors causes impaired digestion, failure to grow, loss of enzymes in the feces, poor health and enlargement of the pancreas. We cannot expect people that work all day to spend much time preparing food. Therefore it is inevitable that there must come a time when tree nuts and other seeds will be sold on the open market in palatable, germinated form. I have said long ago that there is a billion dollars waiting for the man who will go through the prolonged, tedious research to accomplish this, and I will be his first customer. As animal protein becomes scarce, the burgeoning population will be forced to rely upon the protein and fat of tree nuts. The acreage under the trees would remain available for other purposes.

What are some of the difficulties that a person can have on a raw food diet? Could a RAPID change, without a transition period, be dangerous because of the quantity of toxins that the enzymes can release from storage?

An exclusive raw food diet of limited duration for therapeutic purposes, for a person temporarily freed from work, can cause therapeutic reactions which are unpleasant, and sometimes quite violent. They do not occur in every person. The allergist likes to say these reactions are caused by allergy to some food. But that does not account for cases where permanent improvement followed from some chronic ailment. At the Sanitarium the staff considered these therapeutic reactions wholesome, and the patients were disappointed if the reactions failed to come. I refer to spells of prolonged vomiting or sustained diarrhea; prolonged expectoration of phlegm; appearance of boils or skin eruptions. These phenomena would often appear after a raw food diet or fast of suitable duration.

The sanitarium staff at that time knew nothing of food enzymes but I later concluded that the improvement of metabolic enzyme activity occasioned by decreased digestive enzyme action, can be credited with promoting the curative process. This in turn was in response to help from food enzymes or fasting, both of which tend to dry up digestive enzyme activity, giving metabolic enzymes a free and helping hand to engage in the beneficial therapeutic enzyme reactions which you correctly attribute to the digestive action of metabolic enzymes on stored foreign obnoxious substrates, which Dr. Lindlahr used to call morbid matter.

Yes, this eliminative process could become dangerous if it got violent and therefore is hardly a project for management at home. It should be looked upon as a major event in the life of the participant and worthy of institutional care and observation. If the reactions seem to get out of hand and get too violent, it may become necessary to interrupt the therapeutic diet, or break the fast, and after a period of rest, repeat the procedure until there are no further therapeutic reactions. In judging when an interruption is called for, an evaluation of body weight, rate of the pulse, blood pressure, and body temperature is helpful. The fact that this beneficial therapeutic process is not allergic in nature, but is in the realm of a house-cleaning effort, is suggested when we consider that similar reactions sometimes appear after massive enzyme therapy, and at times even after ordinary enzyme supplementation. I am sure that many cases mistakenly described as allergies are in fact instances in which the process is therapeutic and should not be suppressed or contained but encouraged to continue until it exhausts itself.

What percentage of raw to cooked is necessary for body's enzymatic activities to function without the need of introduction of encapsulated enzymes?

I have stated before that a diet containing 75% of raw calories and 25% of cooked calories is a vast improvement over the virtually enzymeless diet.

I have noticed that a diet high in acid, as well as sub-acid fruit can trigger severe acidosis. Are such fruits actually acid in the final effect on the bloodstream or is it the enzymes which release volumes of acids from internal crystallized storage that are responsible for the acidosis? In particular I have noticed severe kidney pains, water retention, acid vomit and urine, and sciatica pains. Vegetables do not seem to produce this effect. Why?

You must remember that not all persons experience the symptoms you mention after use of citrus fruit. On this point it may be instructive to quote from an article I wrote for the July 1925 issue of the *Lindlahr Magazine Of Health*: "Blatherwick has conclusively demonstrated that the organic acids contained in fruits are completely oxidized before leaving the stomach, and the heavy mineral content is then at the disposal of the organism. It has been shown by this investigator that ingestion of liberal amounts of acid fruit renders the urine less acid, and if large quantities are eaten, the urine assumes an alkaline reaction. Herbivorous animals in the suckling stage, and the suckling human infant, have a urine possessing much the same characteristics as that of carnivora. When herbivora or man live on their own tissues, as during a period of starvation or fasting, they become carnivorous, and their urine alters completely in character, corresponding now to the urine of flesh eaters." Comparative physiology teaches that the urine of herbivorous animals is alkaline in reaction.

The report referred to is by W.R. Blatherwick and M.I. Long and appeared in *The Journal of Biological Chemistry*, October 1923, under the title, "Studies of Urinary Acidity". According to my recollection, a group of medical students drank orange juice but I cannot remember how much. They were the subjects upon whom the tests were conducted. If there is a medical school in your city, its library will have the journal mentioned and you can get complete details. It would require much more data than you state to evaluate your symptoms. Most people can tolerate moderate amounts of citrus fruits without symptoms. The use of large amounts of such fruits as a normal permanent diet cannot be accepted because there is no evidence that any species of living organism had used such a diet. There is no indication that any tribe or race of humans, or any species of animal, used large amounts of such fruits every day for extended periods. Therefore, there are no grounds for saying that eating large amounts of acid fruits every day as a normal diet is either good or bad. I have used 2 glasses of fresh citrus fruit juice daily for extended periods, and have seen others drink 3 glasses each day without observing any untoward effects. But in some people even small amounts produce symptoms and in these cases a diagnosis must be made to establish if the symptoms are therapeutic reactions. Citrus fruit is useful in sustaining and therapeutic diets because it offers some food enzymes and high quality sugars which supply "good" calories, as apart from "evil" calories supplied by skeletonized, refined sugar. To Official Chemistry, raw and cooked calories are just calories - having no difference at all on your health and well being. But I take no such promiscuous, carefree and irresponsible attitude toward the health of those eating "damaged" calories.

During fasting there is a reduction in the digestive enzyme production. How is this surplus, as well as that associated with leukocytosis, used by the body during fasting?

Fasting provides a holiday vacation for the digestive enzymes and allows the enzyme potential to devote all of its attention to producing the hundreds of metabolic enzymes needed to run all activities. When you have a two week vacation you have a chance to paint you house, wax your car, fix your roof, or tend to any other neglected chore which must be ignored during the rest of the year. The enzyme potential of the body is under great pressure to keep up the rich enzyme digestive secretions. The only time it gets a breathing spell is during fasting, during a period of exclusive raw food diet, or when supplemental enzymes are used to digest enzymeless food.

Can you comment on the metabolism of seeds during soaking, sprouting, germinating as well as fermenting (when converted to seed or nut milk, and inoculated by airborne bacteria or specialized bacteria) from the point of view of enzymes?

This is taken up in the book *ENZYME NUTRITION*. Germination increases the enzyme activity as much as 6 times. This is due to proteolytic release of the enzymes by inactivation of the enzyme inhibitors found in all seeds. Soaking the seeds allows proteases within to neutralize the inhibitors and release the enzymes from bondage. During the years 1930 to 1940 chemists spoke of free and bound enzymes in seeds. It was found that such proteases and papaine soaked in water with the seeds, released the "sleeping" enzymes from bondage. In 1944 when enzyme inhibitors were discovered in seeds the mystery was cleared up.

Would you consider the behavior of chlorophyll and hemoglobin as being enzymatic?

There is not a single function taking place in any animal or plant organism that is not powered by enzyme action. There are thousands of enzymes at work doing different jobs - one author estimating 100,000. Metabolism is an enzymic process from beginning to end. Metabolism is Mr. and Mrs. Grandparent Enzyme and their children, grandchildren, great grandchildren and all of their offspring and in-laws, multiplied many times, and all of them ceaselessly at work. The most extensive and persistent work on enzymes involved in the metabolism of plants, including chlorophyll, was done at the Laboratory of the Hawaiian Sugar Cane Planters Association on the sugar cane plant.

What is the value of rejuvilac (soaking of wheat in water for 2-5 days) drink as a source of enzymes?

I know nothing about Rejuvilac. About 40 years ago I had a small laboratory in my home and made numerous viscosity enzyme tests on the amylase content of resting and germinated wheat seeds. But it never occurred to me to test the water in which the seeds had been soaked. I believe, however, that most, if not all, of the enzyme activity is retained in the seed, unless the seeds are crushed or mashed and dissolved in the water in the form of a suspension.

Considering that today there are many folks who are living on a totally raw food diet for up to 25 years duration, do you feel inspired by the receptivity of the public to your pioneer work?

I would feel better if these people would spread the word to the millions who do not comprehend the idea.

Compare values of encapsulated plant enzymes and enzymes as found in raw foods, e.g. is a large salad of sprouts, ferments, greens, before a cooked vegetarian meal sufficient to digest the food without the body needing to create additional enzymes in excess of what is available by way of pancreas (that is no leukocytosis after a mixed meal)?

The enzymes in supplements or in digestive secretions are much stronger then in raw foods. But raw foods stimulate the secretion of weaker hydrochloric acid in the stomach and therefore the enzymes in raw foods are able to act for a longer period in the stomach than when cooked food is eaten. Many years ago, when I was making enzyme tests of foods, I did not make enzyme tests on sprouts. I had a preconceived idea that the sprout was a recipient of some of the increase in enzyme activity brought about by germination. The commercial germinators of barley changed my mind. In large plants, tons of barley seeds are kept moist for several days until they germinate. When the sprout reaches no more than a fraction of an inch in length, the enzymes in the seed have multiplied enormously, and the seeds are ready for use. The sprout is discarded because it has been found to have little enzyme activity. Not having made actual tests on bean sprouts, I cannot say how much enzyme activity they have. But in view of the data on barley sprouts I must rate bean sprouts with leafy vegetables and greens as a good source of minerals and vitamins, but relatively poor in enzymes.

Some raw foods contain enzyme inhibitors, especially seeds. How are they effected by fermentation and germination?

From the data in my files it would be proper to say that all seeds contain enzyme inhibitors, while the leaves, stems, roots and the fleshy part of fruits contain no inhibitors. Enzyme inhibitors are inactivated by germination. Since fermentation is an enzymic process, there is reason to believe that it also inactivates enzyme inhibitors.

What are some of the dangers of a macrobiotic diet which relies on mostly cooked grains and other cooked produce?

I am not familiar with the term macrobiotic diet. However, a diet using cooked food forces body enzymes to action and cannot therefore, in the strict sense, be acknowledged to be a healthful diet. The LAW OF THE ADAPTIVE SECRETION OF ENZYMES ordains that the digestive secretions must be kept unphysiologically rich in enzymes in digesting enzymeless cooked food. Because the enzyme potential of the organism is limited, in the course of time, the metabolic enzymes of the body become understaffed, so to speak, because too many enzymes are being sent to the digestive tract. Consequently the metabolism of the whole body suffers. The weakest organ system breaks down first in the form of a local malfunction which may shortly blossom into a disease. Abundant evidence supports this philosophy, but surprisingly, it has not yet been utilized by the writers of texts on physiology and incorporated into these volumes.

Does slow baking at low temperature of root and tubers preserve enzyme content?

Any kind of heat treatment of food in the kitchen destroys 100% of its enzymes. Slow or fast baking, slow or fast boiling, stewing, frying, all destroy 100% of the enzymes in food. Vigorous boiling takes place at 212 degrees F; slow boiling at 190 to 200 degrees. Frying is done at a much higher temperature and in addition to destroying enzymes, it also damages protein, or forms new chemical compounds with unknown, and possibly pathogenic possibilities, imposing still more burden upon the metabolic enzymes. Although baking takes place at 300 to 400 degrees, it is in dry heat, so the destructive effect is no more than at boiling temperatures. Enzymes are completely destroyed at all of these temperatures.

When I was in active practice I developed special electrothermotherapy immersion apparatus to apply high temperature treatment to specific parts of the body to stimulate local enzyme activity which increases 2 to 3 times for every 10 degrees increase in local temperature. I modified some of this apparatus to permit experiments to determine the thermal death point of protoplasm, and found that immersion in water at 118 degrees F destroyed enzymes in 1/2 hour. The temperature of 118 degrees also blistered the skin, and it prevented germination of various seeds when they were immersed for 1/2 hour. Comparing 118 degrees with any of the cooking temperatures, you can see that the enzymes in foods have not the slightest chance of escaping destruction under any kind of kitchen heat exposure.

Do oils or honey in the raw state have any enzyme activity value in one's diet?

Crude, thick, turbid olive oil is a good source of lipase. At one time this kind of olive oil had a good reputation in Spain and Italy. It was used by women on the hair and skin and highly rated. All oils and fats in the natural state contained the enzyme lipase - modern clear oils have none. In human obesity and in human lipomas, lipase is found in smaller amounts. In the book ENZYME NUTRITION, I have shown by extensive documentation that lipase in the diet has a favorable influence in cardiovascular disease by taming cholesterol.

Natural, raw honey has several enzymes, amylase (diastase) being the enzyme best known. It digests starch. In cooler climates extracted honey hardens from a liquid into a solid, opaque mass. This spoils its sales value, so it is heated for as long as 72 hours at pasteurizing (145 degrees F) temperatures. This keeps it clear on the shelves of stores, but unfortunately it destroys its enzymes. Honey has always been famous for its amylase which science has proven comes from pollen and not from the bee. The enzyme was valued highly in Germany and Holland in former times and laws were enacted grading honey according to its enzyme content.

What are your thoughts on urine therapy? I am under the impression that the urine toxins are filtered out by the intestinal tract wall and the body is highly benefited by the recycling of the urine, water soluble vitamins and minerals.

When I maintained groups of albino rats on raw and cooked diets, I made daily tests at certain periods on the amylase output in their urine and feces. Although the enzyme loss is a mere fraction of the tremendous amount of digestive enzymes poured into the digestive canal it is welcomed by plants when it gets into the soil. I have had no experience with autogenous urine therapy, nor have I followed the literature on it.

Do you have any final comments as to how an enzyme rich diet can be used as a tool in this age of ecological crises and technological disasters? Can it protect us from environmental poisons, radiation, and disease?

As I have repeatedly pointed out in writings, keeping up a high enzyme potential is the one way the body has to deal with tobacco smoke, short wave radiation, toxic chemicals, and the prevention and cure of disease. There is no other mechanism in the body except enzyme action to protect the body from any hazard. It is ambiguous to say that nature cures, when we must know that the only machinery in the body to do anything is enzyme action. Hormones do not work. Vitamins cannot do any work. Minerals were not made to do any work. Proteins cannot work. Nature does not work. Only enzymes are made for work. So it is enzymes that cure. Therefore the ability of the body to make any of the numerous enzymes needed for good health and long life must be kept at a high level by the methods incorporated in *The Food Enzyme Concept*.

When George Bernard Shaw reached his zenith years he made some remarks which I must reconstruct according to memory because I do no have the exact words. In effect he said he had been around so long that in due time people will grow weary of seeing ghostly remains of a once imposing G. B. S. wandering hither and thither and some may wish he would fade away and permanently disappear from the scene. Being past eighty, and as energetic as at an earlier age, I feel it would be possible to reach the century mark, had not my body been damaged by early errors in living and unwarranted surgical intervention, as I have explained elsewhere. As it is I do not plan remaining around here for more than a few more years, or until I can be dispossessed of several annoying problems which are begging to be solved.

Thank you very much for sharing these most appropriate and valuable discoveries. I look forward to the day of meeting you in person.

Appendix II
Groundbreaking Research on Enzymes Proves Dramatically Increased Amino Acid and Peptide Absorption at the Cellular Level

A recently completed leading-edge in vitro study has demonstrated that combining a particular proprietary proteolytic enzyme and mineral blend with a certain patented nutraceutical, led to **40% more peptides and amino acids being absorbed into the intestinal cells while also increasing the absorption rates by over 30%.**

The implications of this result means that individuals could potentially benefit from the use of the plant enzymes combined with this specific mineral blend to:

- enhance natural energy
- reduce incidence of food and airborne allergies
- speed up recovery from any illness or injury
- have healthier hair, skin and nails
- burn more calories during digestion
- build muscle mass or maintain muscle tone
- reduce gas, bloating or intestinal discomfort

The complete study is available for review and download at: *http://www.enxymessence.com/research/index.html.*

Viktoras Kulvinskas, M.S.